Everything You Need To Know About Multiple Sclerosis

For MS Warriors, Their Family, Friends and Care Givers

Paul Lima

Every Thing You Need To Know About Multiple Sclerosis
- First Edition 2018

Cover and interior design: Paul Lima. Copyright © 2018

Published by Paul Lima Presents
www.paullima.com/books

Manufactured in the U.S.A.
Published in Canada

ISBN: 978-1-927710-32-6

Dedication

To MS Warriors around the world. Long may you fight!

Contents

1 / Introduction

My name is Paul Lima. I am an MS Warrior. That is what people with MS call themselves as they battle this insidious disease. Three to four million of us are affected by Multiple Sclerosis (MS) worldwide. I have had MS since 1998, for over twenty years as of the writing of this book. There have been years when it has pretty much knocked me on my butt. Years when it has given me strange and bizarre symptoms. Years when it has disappeared to wherever MS goes when those with Relapsing Remitting MS go into remission and, for the last four years, it has knocked me on my butt and kept me from doing all but walking my dog, a Giant Schnauzer named Quinn, and teaching some online writing courses for the University of Toronto. And that is more than many people with MS can accomplish.

During the 20 years that I've had MS, I've learned a lot about this disease. More than I've cared to learn, but it can pay to know your enemy.

I am not a doctor, so this is a layman's guide to MS. I have researched and verified every fact presented, to the best of my ability. And I hope the writing makes the facts presented clear and understandable. Hopefully the fact that I have been a freelance writer, author and writing trainer for the last thirty years helps me do that. (If you want to know more about me, and what I do—or try to do as I deal with my MS—go to paullima.com.)

But this book isn't about who I am and what I am personally dealing with, although I have a chapter about MS and me in this book. This book is about everything (or almost everything) you need to know about MS. From first inklings, or the fact that something strange is going on, to the diagnosis, to what and why MS is, to types of MS, to medications and potential side effects, to diet, exercise and depression, to relationships and more. My hope is that this book will help you understand this chronic disease—to understand that MS is not a death sentence, but that it can have a detrimental impact on your physical and emotional well being. And to understand that MS is different for everybody diagnosed with the disease.

That's right. *Different.* For each MS Warrior. Just like every snowflake is different, there are different types of MS, and there are different symptoms for each person living with MS. But just like every snowflake is made from frozen water, MS Warriors, as we shall see, have similarities too.

I've written this book because I was surprised at how naïve many of the questions asked by those with MS were, and how frightened many of those newly diagnosed with MS seemed to be. Then it occurred to me, after twenty years of dealing with MS, I was a veteran. Twenty years ago, my questions were just as naïve, probably more so. I was just as frightened, even more so.

It's not that I now have all the answers. Not by a long shot. Nobody has all the answers. Nor am I now a big, brave guy! Not at all. But I am no longer new to MS and I have a bit more understanding about MS. Don't get me wrong. MS still scares the crap out of me. I've just learned how to breathe and remain calm in the face of my fears—most of the time.

Yes, your doctors have information. But they can only dispense information in twenty-minute sessions once or twice a year. Unfortunately, much of it, especially if you are newly diagnosed, goes in one ear and out the other and leaves you with more questions than answers. Not the fault of the doctors (in most cases). It's difficult to absorb information when you've been given a *sentence* (formally called a *diagnosis*) that you really don't understand and that scares the crap out of you.

Yes, there is a lot of information online and I encourage people with MS, and their family members and caregivers, to read about MS on legitimate websites (see my list of online resources at the end of this book). I also encourage you to join in-person support groups (check with local chapters of MS societies for information about support groups) and online support groups such as Facebook MS support groups or myMSteam, the social network for those living with MS. At the same time, it seems like there was room, maybe even a need, for a book that catalogues just about everything one needs to know about MS.

With all of that in mind, if you have MS, I hope that it is not severe and that this book gives you some sense of what you might expect to deal with over time. If you are a family member of someone with MS, or caring for some with MS, I hope that this book gives you a greater sense of what the MS Warrior might be going through. In other words, I hope this book helps you feel more prepared for what may come—although I hope it does not arrive for a long, long time.

Suffice it to say, while many MS Warriors have decent days, weeks, months, and even years, they still have a bizarre disease that can manifest itself in different ways at any time. Whatever your case, do not let MS define you. You are not your disease.

Note: I have not sent this book out for editing as I'd normally do. If you see any typos, feel free to email me (msandmebook@mail.com) and I will fix the errors in the next edition.

Paul Lima
February 2019

2 / What Is MS?

People have asked me: Is Multiple Sclerosis (MS) a disease or disability? The answer to that question is both simple and complex. MS is a disease that can be exhausting and debilitating. In other words, MS can lead to disabilities. It can be physically, emotionally and mentally draining an devastating. It can ruin lives and relationships. It can make small tasks incredibly difficult to accomplish. It can put you in a wheelchair chair with legs that won't work and arms that are all but paralyzed. It can leave you so deeply depressed it would take a miracle to lift you out of the deep hole of despair you have fallen into.

But for some MS comes and goes, leaving you able to more or less enjoy a normal life when it disappears. And bowling you over when it decides to again rear its ugly head. In short, MS is erratic and unpredictable.

In this book I will attempt to tell you everything you need to know about MS, but I don't think I can make you feel it, make you feel what MS Warriors feel on their worst days. For that, you need to have MS, which I would not wish on anybody. However, I hope you gain more understanding into what MS is and does to those who have it.

At the same time, you might read about miracle MS cures and recoveries and about people bouncing back from extreme lows with experimental interventions. It happens. You might know people with MS who feel fine or at least more or less all right. You might hear about, or know people with MS, who don't seem physically, mentally or emotionally down and out at all. That too happens and there are reasons for it, which we will go into.

However, MS can be, and too often is, an insidious disease that is different for each person who has it. For many, too many, with MS, it is the worst of times or over time it becomes the worst of times. A few, too few, with MS, experience the best of times. At least as best as it can get if you have a bizarre, inconsistent and incurable disease.

With that in mind, let's look at *what* MS is, so we know what we're talking about, and then get to different types of MS before we look at the *why* of MS.

MS is considered an autoimmune disease in which the body's immune system attacks its own tissues. In the case of MS, this immune system malfunction creates lesions on the brain, spinal cord and/or optic nerve by destroying myelin, the protective sheath or fatty substance that coats and protects nerve fibers. This process is called demyelination and it is this destruction, and the lesions the destruction creates, that cause various types of MS and various MS symptoms.

MS is a long-lasting disease, as in lifelong. It can cause problems with vision, balance, muscle control, and other basic bodily functions, but more on that later. The effects, as I've said, are pretty much different for everyone who has the disease.

Some people with MS experience very little disability during their lifetime. Many experience roller coaster disabilities: they are up and they are down at different times with different symptoms that last varying lengths of times. Some people experience a steady decline in health. Up to sixty per cent of those with MS are no longer fully able to walk twenty years after onset, which has major implications for their quality of life and costs to society.

As I've said, MS is the *Snowflake Disease*. Just like every snowflake is different, MS is different, or mostly different, for every person who has it. And just like every snowflake has some common conditions—created out of frozen water, for instance—every person with MS has some common conditions, such as demyelination that creates lesions and causes the various symptoms.

Lesions, sometimes called scars or plaques, are the hallmarks of MS. They can appear on the brain, spinal cord or optic nerve. Symptoms of MS and its accompanying relapses tend to manifest according to where the disease creates lesions. For example, when a lesion occurs in the optic nerve, vision problems tend to occur. However, there is no one-to-one comparison for how lesions in different areas correspond to specific symptoms.

An *exacerbation* or flare is a time when MS symptoms suddenly start or become worse, generally caused by the onset of new or expanding lesions. Some exacerbations are followed by partial recoveries; some are not, as we will see in the next chapter.

3 / Types of MS

When it comes to MS, people experience body parts falling asleep or having strange tingles, as if being attacked by pins and needles. They experience fatigue, blackouts, dizziness, incontinence, headaches, aching limbs or other body parts. They have issues with balance and/or swallowing. They may have teeth, jaw, vision and/or cognitive dysfunctions. They may be sensitive to heat or to cold, or to both. They might have strange itchiness or they might have tightening around the chest or other body parts. I know people with MS who use canes or walkers, people in wheelchairs, people who can't use their arms, barely use their hands. I could go on. And on…

And then there are people with MS who are perfectly healthy. Until they are not. With that in mind, here is some information on the official four types of MS:

Relapsing-Remitting MS (RRMS). This is the most common type of MS. About eighty-five percent of people with MS are initially diagnosed with RRMS. People with RRMS have temporary periods when new symptoms appear (length and severity varies). These periods are called relapses or exacerbations. And then they have quiet times when all is relatively normal—when the relapse remits or goes away. During the normal times, when symptoms improve, the body heals some of the lesion damage. This is a process known as *remyelination*. Many MS veterans can tell you about recoveries that have been so complete they have simply been able to get on with life as they knew it before their MS diagnosis.

Secondary-Progressive MS (SPMS). In SPMS, symptoms develop and worsen steadily over time, without remissions. The rate at which they occur and become more severe differs for each person with SPMS. Most people, but not all people, who are diagnosed with RRMS transition to SPMS at some point.

Primary-Progressive MS (PPMS). This type of MS occurs in about ten percent of people with MS. PPMS is characterized by symptoms that worsen from the beginning of the development of MS, with no remissions. Sadly, people with PPMS tend to end up using walkers and eventually wheelchairs. They may need help getting in and out of bed and even eating meals and going to the bathroom.

Progressive-Relapsing MS (PRMS). A rare form of MS, PRMS is characterized by a steadily worsening disease state from the beginning, with acute relapses but no remissions. Conditions worsen at a more rapid rate than those who have PPMS.

A new subtype of MS has been identified by researchers. In many ways the discovery changes our understanding of the disease. The newly identified subtype—called myelocortical MS (MCMS)—features a loss of neurons but no damage to the brain's white matter. In other words, no demyelination. The research findings show that neuron loss and demyelination can occur independently in MS and highlights the need for more sensitive MRI scans.

It may be a new subtype of MS but it still leaves people with MS

In addition, there is a school of thought that says **MS is a spectrum**, as opposed to there being four distinct types. Different people with MS are on different places of the spectrum at different times and they progress along the spectrum at different rates.

With all that in mind, let's take a closer look at relapses or flares.

Relapses or Flares

If you have MS but feel fine for months (or even years) but then new MS symptoms pop up or old ones reoccur, you are most likely having what doctors call an exacerbation, relapse or flare.

Flares happen when inflammation in your nervous system damages the myelin that covers and protects nerve cells. This damage slows or stops nerve cell signals from getting to the parts of your body where they need to go.

If you have RRMS, you may have flares followed by symptom-free periods called remissions. To be a true relapse, the symptom must start at least 30 days after your last flare and should stick around for at least 24 hours. Most flares stick around for weeks, months or even a year or so. As discussed, everyone's flare is different. Some are mild. Others are severe.

During a flare you'll get new symptoms, old ones will return or the ones you have will get worse. There is no way to guarantee that you can prevent flares. Disease modifying drugs (DMD) seem to slow MS and help prevent relapses, but DMDs work differently for everybody on them and many have server side effects (but more on drugs coming up).

Staying as healthy as possible, aside from your MS, can help you deal with MS. For instance, a cold or the flu can set off your MS symptoms, so wash your hands frequently, get your yearly flu shot, and avoid hanging around people who have a contagious illness.

If you smoke, quit. It's bad for you in so many ways, and it can make your MS symptoms worse. Talk to you doctor about ways to break the habit.

While it is easier said than done, try to relax. Stress can bring on a relapse so, if needed, try meditation or yoga to help you relax. I don't take well to meditation or yoga but I find reading helps me relax. You need to find your path to relaxation. Again, more on all of this coming up.

In addition to relaxing, rest when you can. Ironically, if fatigue is one of your MS symptoms, resting won't make it go away. Being fatigued is much different from simply feeling tired. When I suffered from fatigue I could get eight hours of sleep, wake up, have breakfast and pass out. When I came to an hour or so later, I'd feel just as exhausted as I did before I passed out.

Unfortunately, people who have never experienced fatigue may think you are simply being lazy when you are, in fact, fatigued. Short of passing out in front of them, I'm not sure what you can do to convince them that you have a disease. You may have to explain to family members, friends and co-worker that you are experiencing fatigue. Tell them what it is and why it is, and hope for the best, which would be an understanding of your debilitating condition.

Having said that, it's still good to be as well rested as you can be. That might help keep other flares at bay. It won't prevent them, but it may help keep you on an even keel. However, all the rest in the world will not thwart your fatigue.

4 / Why Is MS?

According to the Mayo Clinic (I think you would have to agree that the Mayo Clinic is a rather authoritative medical institution): "The cause of multiple sclerosis is unknown."

So much for the *why*. Doesn't make anybody with MS feel any better, but what are you going to do? Make up a reason if the reason is unknown?

However, just because an authoritative voice such as the Mayo Clinic says we don't know what causes MS, and I suspect we really don't, that doesn't prevent people from speculating. In addition, it is known that MS is associated with several factors.

For instance, your chance of developing MS is slightly higher if a close relative, such as a parent or sibling, has the disease. So genetics may have something to do with MS, in some instances. According to the National Multiple Sclerosis Society of America, if one parent or sibling has MS, the chances of another family member getting the disease are approximately 2.5 to 5 percent. Meanwhile, the chances that the average person will get MS are approximately 0.1 percent. So is MS hereditary? Perhaps in some cases seems to be the general consensus.

Epidemiologists have seen an increased pattern of MS in countries located farthest from the equator. In short, MS is far more common in countries with temperate climates, including Canada (the country in which I live), the northern United States, New Zealand, parts of Australia and Europe. This correlation causes some to believe that vitamin D (the sunshine vitamin), or the lack of it, may play a role in why people develop MS.

People who live closest to the equator have the lowest incidences of MS. But put those two factors together and how do you explain why the disease is nearly absent among Canada's Inuit in the High Arctic and among indigenous people in North America and Australia, or why it is rarely found in Japan. So does a vitamin D deficiency cause MS? The jury is still out on this.

Researchers have also considered the possibility that viruses and bacteria may cause MS. Viruses are known to cause inflammation and a breakdown of myelin. Therefore, it's possible that a virus could trigger MS.

In addition, new research suggests that MS starts in the gut. Researchers at the University of Zurich believe that the immune cells are activated in the intestine and then migrate to the brain, where they cause an inflammatory cascade. In the MS patient, T-cells—the white blood cells that help govern the immune system—react to a protein called GDP-L-fucose synthase that's found in bacteria in the gut. In their therapy, the researchers take blood from the MS patient, and then add protein fragments to the surface of the red blood cells in order to re-educate the immune system to tolerate brain tissue, instead of attacking it.

If MS starts in the gut, the discovery might open the door to a therapy that could reverse MS. But don't hold your breath in anticipation of prevention or a cure any time soon!

While MS is most often diagnosed in adults aged 15 to 40 years old, younger children and older adults are also diagnosed with the disease. I was 42 when I had my first known symptoms. In addition, gender might come into play as women are two to three times more likely to develop MS than are men. But nobody knows why gender could be an issue.

We could go on, but the fact is we don't really know why people develop MS or what causes it and why some people with MS react to some things better than others, while some people with MS have adverse reactions to some things that seem to help, or have no real impact on, others. This is something that can be said about many diseases, and many things, in life. So in that respect, I suppose, people with MS are not so special after all. We just think we are!

A more important question, until the cause of MS is determined for certain, might be this: What causes MS to flare up? Again, the jury is still out, but there are some thoughts on what causes MS to flare up.

Emotional stress can lead to the common MS symptom of depression. Stress can also lead to other MS symptoms, such as fatigue and confusion. With that in mind, an important aspect of MS treatment is creating a support network that may include loved ones who can physically help MS Warriors or a support group that can provide emotional strength. People with MS might also want to consider stress-relieving activities such as meditation and yoga.

Fatigue can cause MS symptoms to flare up. While sleep is important for everyone, it's essential for those with MS as most people with MS have a lower reserve of energy.

Infections can be the cause of MS flare ups, such as urinary tract infections. Some people with MS have reduced bladder function making them more susceptible to urinary tract infections. In addition, any infection that weakens the immune system, such as a cold or the flu, can cause a flare.

Heat can cause flares in some people with MS. In others it is not an issue. An infection that leads to a fever can be troublesome as the fever leads to increased body heat. At the same time, hot weather or even hot showers can cause flares. On the other side of the coin, some people with MS do tolerate cold very well or find that cold weather can lead to exacerbations.

In short, there is a lot we don't know for certain about MS and it's cause or the causes of various MS symptoms. The hope is that one day we will know the cause of MS and that knowing the cause will lead to MS prevention and will help scientists find a cure for MS.

But until that day, MS Warriors have little choice but to deal with the hand that they have been dealt.

5 / First Inklings of MS

My MS started with a strange needles and pins tingling in my fingers and hands that spread into my arms and up into my chest and as well as down into my legs. Other than the strange sensation, I felt fine. But with the encouragement of my wife, Lyn, I went to see my doctor.

I didn't know how lucky I was. What I was experiencing seemed like a neurological disorder to my doctor, so he got me to see a neurologist, the person who is responsible for taking you through the tests that lead to a diagnosis of various neurological disorders, including MS.

After a number of tests that I will get into, I was diagnosed with "possible MS." The reason it was called "possible" is that you need at least two flare ups (multiple flare ups) for the diagnosis to be called *multiple* sclerosis. I have since had multiple flare ups and have been officially diagnosed with RRMS, although it seems like I have transitioned into SPMS.

It took about two months, from the strange sensations to seeing the neurologist, to receive my diagnosis. I know people with MS who wait three, four, five, or more years before they get to see a neurologist, let alone get a proper diagnosis. In the vast majority of cases, this is not the fault of the medical industry. Unfortunately, the symptoms these people present are different than mine and do not seem neurological in nature. Hence, their doctors do not send them to see neurologists. In fact, if they had been sent to see a neurologist, he or she would have wondered why the patient was there.

If your symptoms are problems with your vision, it makes sense for your doctor to send you to an eye doctor. If you are having problems with your feet, why wouldn't your doctor send you to podiatrist? Bladder issues? There is a specialist you should see. Pains in your joints? Spasms? General fatigue? Balance problems? Dizziness? Cognitive problems? There are specialists who examine people with such issues.

Now most people with MS have some of these symptoms at some point in the progression of their disease. But if these symptoms are the first ones that you have, you will most likely not be sent to a neurologist, the one person who can run the tests required for you to be diagnosed with MS.

Just to be clear, I am not saying that if you have some of the symptoms I've mentioned that you have MS. I am saying if you have MS and you present with symptoms not typically associated with a neurological disorder, it may take a while—until you have other symptoms—before you get to see a neurologist and get a proper diagnosis.

Remember how I called MS the Snow Flake disease? MS presents itself differently for almost everyone who gets this bizarre illness. Why did my MS initially manifest itself in ways that seemed as if it could be a neurological issue? Why is it that someone else with MS may have initial eye issues that are not diagnosed as MS-related optic neuritis? It does so because MS is such a weird and whacky disease.

However, a more medical answer may be that it depends on where the lesions are on your brain, spine or optic nerve. For instance, if you have lesions on your optic nerve causing you eye issues, you doctor does not know that lesions are at the root of your symptoms. It takes an MRI to detect that, and typically you have to be sent to a neurologist to be booked for an MRI. So your general practitioner, who you have gone to with eye issues, or fatigue, or memory loss, or bladder problems and so on, will send you to the appropriate specialist and you will be misdiagnosed—through no fault of the doctors who are diagnosing you.

So your first inklings may not lead to a proper diagnosis. I was diagnosed with RRMS after my second flare up.

But even once you've had MS, you can have ailments that are not attributed to MS. For instance, I know MS Warriors who have had sever jaw pain and have been diagnosed with trigeminal neuralgia, a condition that's most commonly caused by nerve compression on the trigeminal nerve that provides sensation to a large portion of the face, including the upper and lower jaws. Some of these people have had root canals and other treatments and the issue has not cleared up. Guess why? The issue was caused by an MS flare up, but they had been feeling fine before the flare up and nobody thought of MS as the cause of the issue.

6 / Doctors & Diagnosis

As we have seen, testing for MS is complex. According to the Mayo Clinic, there are no specific tests for MS. Instead, a diagnosis of MS relies on ruling out other conditions that might produce similar signs and symptoms. That often makes the path to a diagnosis of MS long and uncertain.

As mentioned, mine was relatively quick, although it was initially for "possible" MS. I needed that second flare for it to be true MS, and that took a couple of years—not that I'm complaining about time between flares.

For some, years may pass between experiencing the first symptoms and receiving an MS diagnosis. Other conditions may be suspected or incorrectly diagnosed before a person is finally diagnosed with MS. Unfortunately, some people have multiple chronic conditions, making it even more difficult for doctors to identify MS.

Compounding all of that, as mentioned, there is no one test that proves MS. Instead, there are three main criteria, all of which must be present for a person to be diagnosed with MS:

Evidence of damage in at least two separate parts of the central nervous system (CNS), which includes the brain, spinal cord, and optic nerves

Evidence that the CNS damage happened at different or multiple times

Every other possible condition must be ruled out.

Some medical exams and tests can provide proof of MS-like damage, while others are performed to rule out other conditions that can cause MS-like damage. At the same time, a clearer picture may emerge from a person's medical history and will help a doctor assess factors that may strengthen the suspicion of MS or rule out other conditions.

Neurological exam: The doctor will carefully examine your eyes and reflexes for signs of nerve damage. You will be asked to move your arms and legs in specific ways to test for weakness or lack of coordination. The doctor will test for loss of sensation by touching various parts of your body with a vibrating tuning fork and both sharp and dull items. The neurological exam provides an objective assessment of signs and symptoms that may suggest MS or another condition.

Magnetic resonance imaging (MRI): The MRI is one of the most valuable tools used in diagnosing MS. An MRI uses a strong magnetic field and radio waves to measure the relative water content in the tissues of the CNS. Some types of MRIs incorporate an intravenous injection of gadolinium, or contrast fluid. MRI scans provide the most detailed non-invasive view of the CNS available.

An MRI is painless, but the machine can be loud and bother people who are claustrophobic. You will be asked to report any metal content in your body—pacemaker devices, orthopedic hardware, shrapnel—so the doctor can ensure your safety during the procedure and you might be asked to wear earplugs to diminish the noise.

MRI scans can show the location, extent, and number of lesions on the brain, spinal cord, and optic nerve. Some types of MRIs can differentiate between new lesions, ones that are growing and older damage that has not completely disappeared

Most MS diagnoses are based in large part on MRI results. After a diagnosis of MS is made, most people continue to receive regular MRI scans to track how quickly the disease is progressing or the impact of disease modifying medications meant to slow down the progression of the disease (more on DMDs below).

Evoked potentials (EP): The EP test measures electrical activity in the brain in response to specific stimuli. During an EP test, wires are placed on the scalp in certain areas. The doctor or nurse will then provide stimuli such as light, sound, or physical sensations as the test records brain activity, checking for areas where electrical conduction is slower due to demyelination. EP tests are painless and can help confirm MS by revealing the extent of lesions that may not be detectable by other tests.

Cerebrospinal fluid (CSF) analysis: The CNS is bathed in a liquid called cerebrospinal fluid. It cushions and protects the brain and spinal cord, circulates nutrients and removes waste from the CNS. CSF analysis is a useful tool in diagnosing many neurological conditions.

CSF is collected via **lumbar puncture**, also called an LP or spinal tap. During a lumbar puncture, you will be asked to lie on your side with your knees pulled up to your chest to create space between vertebrae. The doctor or nurse will clean an area over the spine in your lower back and insert a hollow needle between two vertebrae in the spinal canal, the space where the spinal cord is located. They will draw out a small amount of CSF and then bandage the puncture site.

Lumbar punctures can be uncomfortable or painful. You may need to lie down for a while after the LP and avoid strenuous activities for the rest of the day. Some people have headaches or backaches after the procedure, but they are generally fine within a day or two, if not sooner.

In most people with MS, CSF analysis will show evidence of elevated levels of antibodies and proteins called oligoclonal bands. In some people with MS, another type of protein created by the breakdown of myelin is also present. While finding these substances indicates an autoimmune condition, the findings are not conclusive for MS.

You need all of these procedures because dozens of other conditions can produce MS-like symptoms. All of these potential diseases must be ruled out in order to confirm MS. The process of ruling out similar conditions is referred to as differential diagnosis.

Conditions that resemble MS may include brain tumors, nutritional deficiencies, structural damage to the brain or spinal cord, infections such as Lyme disease, syphilis, and HIV, autoimmune disorders such as lupus or Sjögren's syndrome and inherited conditions such as mitochondrial disease.

All of that is why the average patient waits about two years, and often longer, from the time of their first symptoms until they are correctly diagnosed with MS.

So what is the problem if you are diagnosed with MS and it turns out you have, say, Lyme disease? Unfortunately, MRI scans for both MS and Lyme diseases appear similar. If it is thought that you have MS you may be put on drugs to help you combat the disease. Many of the MS DMDs cause various side effects and they can cost a small fortune. In addition, you won't be treated for Lyme disease, which is curable with antibiotics. However, the immunosuppressant drugs that many MS patients are given will worsen Lyme disease. Hence all the tests are necessary.

7 / MS Symptoms

Multiple sclerosis is very rarely a fatal condition. For the most part, people with MS enjoy longevity close to that of people without MS. On average, the lifespan of a person with MS is about seven years shorter than that of others. Most people with MS die of the same conditions other people die of, such as cancer and heart disease. It is only in severe cases of MS, with very rapid progression, that MS is the cause of death, or leads to symptoms that cause death.

Having said that, there are many MS-related symptoms—almost as many symptoms as there are people with MS.

What causes MS symptoms?

As mentioned, MS attacks myelin, the protective covering of the brain, spinal cord and often the optic nerve. This causes inflammation and often damages the myelin in patches (creates what are known as lesions). When this happens, the usual flow of nerve impulses is interrupted or distorted. The result may be the wide variety of MS symptoms, depending upon which parts of the central nervous system are affected. Not all people with MS will experience all symptoms; often the symptoms will improve during periods of remission, although not all those who have MS go into remission. Sadly, some people, those with PPMS, start to, and continue to, deteriorate physically.

Common symptoms

Fatigue occurs in about 80% of people with MS. It can significantly interfere with the ability to function at home and work, and may be the most prominent symptom in a person who otherwise has minimal limitations. When I say "fatigue" I am not talking about just being tired, although that too is an issue. I am talking about an exhaustion so deep that you have no choice but to pass out, as I experienced for about two years before my fatigue symptom went into remission.

Walking difficulties frequently occur, forcing MS Warriors to use canes, walkers, scooters or even wheel chairs. These difficulties tend to be related to factors such as weakness in the legs, spasticity, loss of balance, sensory deficit and fatigue. Often they can be mitigated to various degrees by physical therapy, assistive therapy and medications, but not always. Those with PPMS end up in wheelchairs. I use a cane and know many, too many, MS Warriors who uses some kind of device to assist with mobility.

Spasticity, or the feelings of stiffness and involuntary muscle spasms, can occur in any limb, but it is much more common in the legs.

Numbness or **tingling** of the face, body, or extremities (arms and legs) is often the first symptom experienced by those eventually diagnosed with MS. Like many symptoms, it comes and goes, recurring for different lengths of time.

General weakness in those with MS results from damage to nerves that stimulate muscles. It may often be managed with rehabilitation strategies and the use of mobility aids and other assistive devices. However, not all those with MS respond to treatment.

Vision problems, or **optic neuritis**, can be the first MS symptom for many people, but of course not for all people with MS. Onset of blurred vision, poor contrast vision and pains when one is moving the eyes can be frightening and are often mistaken for eye issues until one is properly evaluated and diagnosed with MS.

Dizziness and **vertigo** frequently affect those with MS, causing them to feel off balance or lightheaded or sometimes creating the sensation that they or their surroundings are spinning. I've had a severe version of this sensation and can tell you that it is not at all fun. Mind you, none of the MS symptoms are any fun.

Bladder dysfunction, which occurs in about 80% of people with MS, can usually be managed successfully with medications, fluid management, and intermittent self-catheterization.

Bowl dysfunction is sometimes a symptom. Constipation is a particular concern among people with MS, as is loss of control of the bowels. Bowel issues can typically be managed through diet, adequate fluid intake, physical activity and medication. But sometimes you have no choice but to go at the most awkward times.

Pain syndromes are common in MS. In one study, 55% of people with MS had "clinically significant pain" at some time, and almost half had chronic pain. For instance, many people with MS experience trigeminal neuralgia, or facial pain (often associated with the jaw or gums). It is a chronic pain condition that affects the trigeminal nerve, which carries sensation from your face to your brain.

My MS pain manifests itself as a constant (24/7 with no relief over the last four years as of the writing of this book) headache. I've tried three medications to combat it, with no success. My neurologist is taking about trying Botox injections next. If the headache does not disappear, I hope that at least some of my wrinkles do!

Some people experience what is known as the **MS hug**. It is an MS symptom where you feel as if you have a tight band around your chest or ribs or it can be pressure on just one side of your torso. Some people find that the MS hug makes it painful to breathe, something that is rather vital I think we'd all agree.

Any pain in the chest needs to be checked by a doctor because it could be some kind of heart or breathing issue. At the same time, if you have already been diagnosed with the MS hug, and a doctor has cleared you of heart issues and the pain returns, you are most likely being hugged again by MS. Still, you need to get it checked out just in case it is not MS. Such is the nature of this bizarre disease.

Some people experience symptoms similar to the MS hug but in their hands or feet, where it feels as though they are constantly wearing gloves or boots. For others, the tight feeling occurs around the head—like wearing a headband that is two sizes too small. The feeling can range from annoying to painful. Others with MS are never hugged at all, other than in sympathy by family and friends.

Some people with MS are **sensitive to heat**, some are **sensitive to cold**. Heat sensitivity is more common and heat can actually cause exacerbations or symptoms to intensify or flare up. Elevated body temperatures in those with MS who have eye issues can further impair vision. This occurs because of damage to the optic nerve that interferes with the transmission of signals between the eyes and the brain

Sexual responses in those with MS can be limited by damage in the central nervous system, as well by symptoms such as fatigue and spasticity, and by psychological or emotional factors.

Cognitive difficulties, a range of high-level brain functions, affect more than 50% of people with MS. Difficulties include the ability to process incoming information, retaining and remembering information, learning new information, organizing and problem-solving, focusing attention and accurately perceiving one's environment.

Fatigue and cognitive issues, not physical disabilities, are the biggest factors that determine whether someone with MS will be able to continue working, or function independently at home. In other words, you can use assistive devices to overcome mobility challenges, but it is much more difficult to maintain employment if you are blacking out from fatigue or if you have difficulty multi-tasking, absorbing or retaining new information or following discussions at meetings. Just like physical difficulties, cognitive issues present differently in each person experiencing them. And, like physical issues, cognitive issues may come and go.

"May" is the operative word, because MS can cause the brain to atrophy, or shrink, which can cause more permanent cognitive dysfunction.

Emotional changes can be a reaction to the stresses of living with MS as well as the result of neurological issues. Significant depression, mood swings, irritability and episodes of uncontrollable laughing and crying pose significant challenges for people with MS.

Studies have suggested that **clinical depression**, the severest form of depression, is a common symptoms of MS. Mind you, if you had to cope with the symptoms described above, often with many of them simultaneously and for prolonged periods of time, you would probably become depressed too. Depression is more common among people with MS than it is in the general population or in persons with many other chronic conditions.

There are also odd issues that only happen on rare occasions and are not categorized. One of my most bizarre MS hits was to the taste buds. I didn't lose my taste. That would have been a blessing in comparison to what happened. What happened was this: everything that I tasted, tasted liked *crap*. Okay, I've never actually tasted crap, so let me qualify that. Everything that I tasted, tasted like what I imagine crap must taste like.

When I say everything, I mean *everything*. Give me a glass of water and I'd say, "Did you draw this water from a polluted swamp?" It was that bad.

I think I lost about thirty pounds while my taste buds were wonky, not that I couldn't stand to lose a few pounds. A couple of months later, all was fine with my taste, and I've managed to keep most of the weight off!

For those with RRMS, symptoms come and go. They may last weeks, months or even years. For those with SPMS, symptoms, for the most part, come and stay. They may pile up over the years. And most unfortunately, those with PPMS experience a slow (and on occasion rapid) decline in mobility and general health.

Less common symptoms

People with MS may experience speech problems, including slurring and loss of volume. This occurs particularly later in the disease and during periods of extreme fatigue. Stuttering is occasionally reported as well.

Swallowing problems, known as dysphagia, result from damage to the nerves controlling the many small muscles in the mouth and throat.

Tremors, or uncontrollable shaking, can occur in various parts of the body because of damaged areas along the complex nerve pathways that are responsible for the coordination of movements.

Seizures, the result of abnormal electrical discharges in an injured or scarred area of the brain, have been estimated to occur in 2 to 5% of people with MS. This compares to the estimated 3% of the general population.

Respiration or breathing problems occur in people whose chest muscles have been severely weakened by damage to the nerves that control those muscles.

Itching is one of the family of abnormal sensations that might be experienced by people with MS.

Although **headaches** are not a common symptom of MS (as mentioned, constant headaches are what I am currently experiencing), some reports suggest that people with MS have an increased incidence of certain types of headaches.

About 6% of people who have MS complain of impaired hearing. In rare cases, hearing loss has been reported as the first symptom of the disease.

Other symptoms

While the symptoms described above are the direct result of damage to the myelin and nerve fibers in the central nervous system, additional symptoms are can arise as a result of the primary symptoms.

For instance, bladder dysfunction can cause repeated urinary tract infections. Inactivity can result in loss of muscle tone as well as overall weakness, poor postural alignment, decreased bone density (resulting in an increased risk of fracture), and inefficient breathing. Immobility can lead to pressure sores.

Some symptoms for those with MS can include social, vocational and psychological complications. For instance, if you are no longer able to drive or walk, you may not be able to hold down your usual job. The stress and strain of dealing with MS often alters social networks and sometimes fractures relationships. I know people with MS who have been deserted by partners, family members and friends. However, I know others who have received amazing support from those around them.

Depression is common in people with MS. It may be a primary symptom as it can be caused by how the disease progresses. However, it can also be triggered by the challenges those with MS face on a daily basis.

There are a variety of ways to try to manage symptoms, ranging from pharmacological treatments to non-medicinal strategies such as physiotherapy, occupational therapy, exercise programs and diet. The problem is that many treatments are not effective for many with MS. And many medical treatments have side effects for some, not all, that can be as bad as, or worse than, the disease. But we will look at that in greater detail in the chapter on medication.

Coming on Fast, Slow, Fast…

MS symptoms often come on fast. One day you're fine, and the next day you have a pins and needles sensation attacking your body. Or all of a sudden you go from an intelligent, articulate individual to one with bizarre cognitive difficulties. Or you have sudden vision problems or ambulatory issues or a tightening around your chest or unexplained headaches or other issues.

On the other hand, symptoms sometimes start slowly. You have minor leg pains or a tightening in your legs that won't go away. A couple of years later you are walking with a cane. A few years later you need a walker. Then a couple of years after that you are using a scooter. A couple of years later you are in a wheelchair.

An acquaintance of mine had PPMS. It took a few years, but slowly his legs started to give out. At first he was still able to walk his dog, but soon he was using a scooter to do so. A couple of years after his dog had passed away and he was pushing himself in a wheelchair. A few years later he was using an electric wheelchair because his arms were weakening and he was not able to push himself around anymore

As I've said, MS is different for all of us. The sad and bizarre fact is that there is nothing normal about MS in the conventional sense of a disease, as in "this is the illness you have, these are the symptoms associated with it, here is the medication you take to combat your disease." MS is one inconsistent, confusing disease. That's why you have to get the various symptoms that may be occurring checked out by your GP, neurologist or some other medical specialist—just in case the symptoms are not MS-related. It's absolutely nuts! But it is the reality of MS.

In short, if you have RRMS and are experiencing an exacerbation, I suggest you use the mantra: "This too shall pass." That doesn't mean you should avoid medications or that you shouldn't try to otherwise deal with your symptoms. That doesn't mean you won't experience pain and discomfort. It means you live your life as best you can, and sometimes it won't be very comfortable, while experiencing the exacerbation, and you focus on the future—when the exacerbation diminishes or disappears—as it often does. It's kind of like looking forward to sunshine on a rainy day.

8 / MS and Medication

As mentioned, MS relapses are caused by inflammation in the central nervous system that damages the myelin coating around nerve fibers. This damage slows or disrupts the transmission of nerve impulses and causes the symptoms of MS. Many relapses, but not all (depending on the type of MS that you have) will gradually resolve without treatment. But many, over time, will not go away. All this begs the question: Should someone with MS take drugs to help combat the disease?

Treatment with DMDs is supported by the MS Coalition which includes the National MS Society. The American Academy of Neurology (AAN) has developed guidelines for starting, switching and stopping DMDs for adults with RRMS. The National MS Society and Multiple Sclerosis Association of America have endorsed these guidelines. According to these agencies, adhering to your DMD is a key element of effective treatment. However, there those who disagree. They say you should use diet to combat MS. Or they point out that many of the potential side effects can be as debilitating as the disease.

I have spent considerable time in various MS forums and have seen people swear that drugs have modified their disease in a positive manner or have helped them combat various symptoms. And I have seen people swear that drugs have cause greater physical or emotional inflictions than the disease.

One MS Warrior put her decision to take drugs this way: "I am more scared of what MS is capable of doing to me left untreated than I am of any potential side effects of the drugs used to treat it. One new lesion in a bad location has the potential to cause devastating disability." With that in mind, she will take prescribed medication in the hope it will keep her exacerbations at bay and allow her to spend more healthy time with her children.

At the same time, somebody I know was on Aubagio, an FDA approved drug. If you go on the pill you have to go in for blood work once a month for the first few months you are on it. You need to have your blood checked to see how your liver is doing. The second time she had her blood tested she did a bit of shopping on her way home. By time she got home there was a message on her answering machine: "Stop taking the pill immediately!"

I know people with MS who feel that their DMDs are helping them cope with the disease. I know people with MS who have moved from drug to drug due to adverse reactions, with no noticeable benefits. I personally have not taken any DMDs and my last two MRIs were what my neurologist would have expected had I been on a DMD. At the same time as my MRIs are improving without drugs, my MS seems to have transitioned from RRMS to SPMS.

In short, it's all a bit of a crapshoot as not every person with MS has the same reaction to the same drug. I am not trying to scare anybody with these stories. I am trying to present common knowledge information. So if you have MS and your neurologist suggests that you take a particular medication, discuss any potential pros and cons with the doctor and make an informed choice. If you take a medication, make sure you are monitored for positive, and potentially negative, developments and make an informed decision to continue with, or to discontinue, the medication. In short, all you can do is refuse treatment and hope that your flare ups are minimal or try the suggested treatment and monitor your reaction to it.

Of course you can also try to tackle your MS with diet and exercise, which we will soon look at.

There are two basic type of MS medications: DMDs meant to increase the time between relapses and decrease their severity of relapses, and drugs you might take to combat various symptoms caused by flare ups.

In recent years, more than a dozen DMDs have successfully been put through clinical trials and have been approved in the United States by the Food and Drug Administration (FDA) based on clinical evidence that they can reduce the number and intensity of lesions, reducing MS flares and slowing the progress of the disease.

Approved DMDs

Injectable medications include: Avonex, Betaseron, Copaxone, Extavia, Glatiramer Acetate Injection, Glatopa, Plegridy and Rebif.

Oral medications include: Aubagio, Gilenya and Tecfidera.

Infused medications (administered intravenously, but may be provided through intramuscular injections and epidural routes into the membranes surrounding the spinal cord) include: Lemtrada, Novantrone, Tysabri and Ocrevus (which is the first medication that is used for some people with PPMS).

Possible Side Effects

Beta interferons are among the most commonly prescribed medications to treat MS. They are injected under the skin or into muscle and can reduce the frequency and severity of relapses. Side effects of beta interferons may include flu-like symptoms and injection-site reactions. You'll also need blood tests to monitor your liver enzymes because liver damage is a possible side effect of interferon use.

Ocrevus is the only DMD approved by the FDA to treat both the RRMS and PPMS. Clinical trials showed it reduced relapse rate in relapsing disease and slowed worsening of disability in both forms of the disease. The drug is given via an intravenous infusion by a medical professional. Side effects may include infusion-related reactions such as irritation at the injection site, low blood pressure, fever, and nausea. Ocrevus may also increase the risk of some types of cancer, particularly breast cancer.

Copaxone may help block your immune system's attack on myelin and must be injected beneath the skin. Side effects may include skin irritation at the injection site.

Tecfidera, a twice-daily oral medication, can reduce relapses. Side effects may include flushing, diarrhea, nausea and lowered white blood cell count.

Gilenya is a once-daily oral medication that reduces relapse rates. You'll need to have your heart rate monitored for six hours after the first dose because your heartbeat may be slowed. Other side effects may include headaches, high blood pressure and blurred vision.

Aubagio is a once-daily medication that can reduce relapse rates. It can cause liver damage, hair loss and other side effects. It is harmful to a developing fetus and should not be used by women who may become pregnant and are not using appropriate contraception.

Tysabri is designed to block the movement of potentially damaging immune cells from your bloodstream to your brain and spinal cord. This medication increases the risk of a viral infection of the brain called progressive multifocal leukoencephalopathy in some people.

Lemtrada helps reduce relapses of MS by targeting a protein on the surface of immune cells and depleting white blood cells. This effect can limit potential nerve damage caused by the white blood cells, but it also increases the risk of infections and autoimmune disorders.

Someone in an MS support forum was diagnosed with RRMS at age 48. It quickly progressed to SPMS and he began to look in earnest for a treatment most likely to stop him from ending up dependent and in nursing care in very short order. His treatment choice was **hematopoietic stem cell transplantation** (HSCT), the transplantation of multipotent hematopoietic stem cells, usually derived from bone marrow, peripheral blood or umbilical cord blood. He is not cured of MS but the treatment seems to have halted the progression of his MS.

HSCT attempts to "reboot" the immune system, which is responsible for lesions in the brain and spinal cord. In HSCT for those with MS, the person being treated is given some form of chemotherapy, usually by infusion in the vein, for up to 10 days to stimulate the production of bone marrow stem cells. Then some blood is drawn from a vein and the stem cells in the blood are stored for later use. The patient is hospitalized and given a powerful mix of chemotherapies for up to 10 days to kill or suppress immune cells throughout the body. The stored stem cells are then infused into the bloodstream through a vein and the individual is given antibiotics to help combat infection.

So will HSCT work for all MS Warriors?

You can read some great testimonials about its effectiveness online. However, HSCT results vary, like the results of all MS medications and diets, so I don't want to be giving false hope by telling you of a treatment that has worked for some, not all, MS Warriors. In addition, as of the writing of this book, the treatment is not approved for use in America or Canada and it is quite expensive.

In fact, in America, the FDA has started to crack down on unscrupulous organizations peddling bogus or unproven—and in some cases dangerous—stem cell treatments. The agency has formed a working group to pursue clinics through whatever legally enforceable means necessary to protect the public health. In other words, stem cell treatments are not without risk. A recent review of safety incidents following use of unproven stem cell treatments found a number of cases of serious complications following treatments. At least 10 treatments resulted in death and 18 resulted in neurological complications. Approved stem cell treatments are being monitored in the US, Sweden, and England.

According to HealthDay News, a stem cell transplant may help some people with MS when standard drugs fail. A relatively new clinical trial focused on 110 patients with aggressive cases of MS: Their symptoms had flared up at least twice in the past year despite taking standard medication, and they'd already tried an average of three of those drugs.

Over an average of three years, MS progressed in 34 of 55 patients on medication, meaning their disabilities worsened. That compared with only three of 55 patients given a stem cell transplant. However, only a small minority of MS patients would be possible transplant candidates. And for now, only certain medical centers have the necessary experience and expertise to perform such transplants.

Bottom line, there are many MS medications and some treatments out there. None of them are a cure for MS. At best, they hold MS at bay, sometimes with no side effects, sometimes with mild side effects and sometimes with excruciating ones. At worse, they do nothing to hold back MS and the side effects are devastating. Some work for some people with MS, but not for others. As I said, it's a crapshoot. Only you can, in consultation with your medical practitioner, can decide if you want to take it.

Drugs to Manage Symptoms

There are a wide variety of medications used to help manage the symptoms of MS, such as bladder problems, bowel dysfunction, infection, depression, dizziness and vertigo, fatigue, various pains in various places, spasticity, tremors and walking (gait) difficulties.

The medications vary, depending on the MS symptoms that are manifesting. You will have to discuss which medications may be appropriate, if any, with your neurologist. For instance, medications such as potent steroids ease inflammation and are often used to treat acute MS exacerbations or relapses.

Someone I know went from walking to a cane to a walker in rather quick succession. His neurologist prescribed a heavy dose of steroids. Five days into taking his meds, his face swelled up like a balloon. Weeks later, he was still using his walker. Does that mean steroids don't work? It means in this instance they didn't work for him. Why? I don't know. You have to ask MS! And you won't get any answers.

In addition, not all relapses need treatment because, as discussed, many, not all, symptoms gradually improve on their own over time. In some instance, steroids or other medications can help the relapse symptoms improve more quickly than it might on its own. In many instance, the medications do nothing or they cause debilitating side effects.

With all of that in mind, my advice is to have an open mind, do your due diligence and make an informed decision about the treatment you consider. Check the facts, in consultation with your neurologist, about which treatments to try and which ones to avoid and make an informed decision.

To sum up, I know people with MS who are on medication that they hope will reduce the size and the number of their lesions and prevent new ones from developing. I know people who are combating their MS with diet. I know people who are taking medication to combat symptoms of MS, as opposed to the MS itself. I know people who have gotten deep brain massages to combat MS and its various symptoms. I know people who are using neuro-acupuncture treatment to combat MS symptoms. And I know people who are doing nothing.

These people all have one thing in common. They all have MS. And it's not going away. But they are doing what they feel may work best for them and their condition because there is no silver bullet that can exterminate this disease or its symptoms. I mean if there was one thing that was working for people with MS, everybody with MS would be doing it. But there isn't one thing. There is no one medication. No one treatment. No one diet. No one routine. No one exercise. No one way of living. No one anything. So you have to decide for yourself, in consultation with your medical practitioners, what you can and should, or should not, do.

Just beware of miracle cures and snake oil salesmen. Because they are out there. They feed off desperate people. They feed us dreams, take our cash, and don't give a hoot if we live or die. You don't have to have MS to meet con artists. History books are full of them.

9 / Grazing in the Grass

We've talked about pharmaceutical medications, now let's talk about… pot, weed, ganga, dope, reefer, Mary Jane, grass—yes, *marijuana*—for a moment.

I want to reiterate that to use drugs or not to use drugs is a personal choice, a lot depending on the type of MS that you have, how severe it is, the symptoms you are dealing with and what your doctor recommends. If you feel a drug can help you, try it and monitor what it is doing and how it is making you feel. That is my attitude when it comes to marijuana too.

I had read that people with chronic illnesses, including MS, were using medical marijuana to manage pain and other symptoms, so I gave it a try. A friend gave me a bit of grass. Thinking about smoking it made my lungs ache (I had bronchitis when I was a kid). However, another friend said she could turn the grass into cannabutter or cannabis-infused butter, and used the cannabutter to make chocolate chip cookies that I could eat.

Now there is something that I did not know about ingesting marijuana. When you smoke it, you get high fairly quickly. When you eat it, it takes about forty-five minutes to get high. I ate one cookie. It seemed to have no effect. So fifteen minutes later, I had a second cookie. I was watching the a mystery thriller TV series at the time. The two cookies kicked in part way through an episode. To this day I have no idea what went on in that episode!

Anyway, the long and the short of it is this: I got high; the MS headaches that I am experiencing did not go away. I tried the cookies several more times, only eating one at a time so that I got much less stoned; the headaches still did not go away.

Marijuana did not work for my condition but I know people with MS who smoke, vape or ingest marijuana on a regular basis. They say it helps them relax, forget about their symptoms or generally feel better. I know people who use medical marijuana with low levels or no levels of Tetrahydrocannabinol (THC), the principal psychoactive ingredient of cannabis. They don't use marijuana to get high but they find they get some relief from it. It simply seems to calm them down and/or calm down their symptoms.

Some people take Cannabidiol, or CBD, a cannabis oil derived from marijuana or industrial hemp. It allegedly relieves pain and inflammation. I say "allegedly" because some people swear by it and others say it has little or no effect. All you can do is try it, monitor the results and make a personal decision.

You also want to be aware of the laws around marijuana in your country or community. I live in Canada where the prescribed use of medical marijuana has been legal for some time and the use of marijuana is now legal (effective October 2018).

In the USA, the medical use of cannabis is legal (with a doctor's recommendation) in 30 or more states, the District of Columbia and the territories of Guam and Puerto Rico. Sixteen other states have laws that allow access to products that are rich in CBD, with limits on the THC content. As of the writing of this book, the recreational use of cannabis is legal in nine states (Alaska, California, Colorado, Maine, Massachusetts, Nevada, Oregon, Vermont, and Washington) and the District of Columbia. Another 13 states plus the U.S. Virgin Islands have decriminalized the use of marijuana.

On an MS support forum one person, who lives with her husband in Central Arkansas, wrote the following about her husband, who has MS:

"I've seen my husband change literally overnight with the use of CBD products. He has sensations in his legs again. In his feet too! He could finally feel that his feet were tired at work last night. Today he carried things in both hands and navigated the living room without balancing himself on anything. His mood has improved. I can't tell you the night-and-day difference CBD has made. I'm not trying to hock a product. I'm just saying that my husband has had major improvements, so much so that I'm sitting here with him looking to find new things for him to do. I cannot believe the difference. If this is what CBD products can do for my husband, then I'm on board. For the first time since all this started happening I feel optimistic. Cautiously optimistic, but optimistic. I'm sitting here laughing to myself thinking, dang, maybe I need to use some CBD oil just to help me with the anxiety I've been dealing with over my husband and his MS."

So just because I didn't have a great experience with marijuana, I would never say don't try it or related products. If you can get some relief from your MS, then good for you. I wish marijuana cookies had worked for me for two reasons: I'd really like to get rid of these freaking headaches and I really enjoyed the chocolate chip cookies!

In short, if you are able to legal try marijuana or CBD oil, do so and see if it helps you better deal with your symptoms in any way.

10 / To MRI or Not To MRI?

MRIs reveal the inside of the brain, eye, and spinal cord in a painless, non-invasive method. While X-rays and computed tomography (CT) scans provide some detail about bones and various body tissues, an MRI reveals much more detail about tissue, showing both the normal structure of the brain and spinal cord, as well as the presence of lesions, scars, or tumors.

In addition to diagnosis, the MRI can aid prognosis (predicting the likely course of one's disease) and disease management. For instance, the number of lesions on an MRI, their location and their size can predict the severity of MS. The location of lesions impact treatment choices and whether the risks of a specific treatment outweigh the benefits.

Once someone with MS starts taking a disease-modifying drug, a periodic MRI assesses whether the treatment is working. It can take six months or so for the drug to produce results so one should not have an MRI right after starting a drug. If the MRI detects new lesions six months or so after one starts taking a drug, then the MRI demonstrates that the individual may not be responding well to the treatment and a treatment change may be in order. In short, an MRI can help with diagnosis, prognosis and monitoring the response to treatment.

Often an MRI will be done with contrast. In other words, MRI images are created after a contrast dye has been injected into the patient's vein. The contrast travels through the bloodstream and into the blood vessels in the brain and spinal cord. These vessels can be seen clearly on an MRI after the contrast has been injected. If active inflammation in the brain or spinal cord with a lesion is taking place at the time of the MRI, the blood vessels near the lesion will be "leaky." Blood vessels become leaky so that white blood cells and other responses to injury can get into the damaged tissue.

There are no known side effects of an MRI scan. However, patients with artificial heart valves, metallic ear implants, bullet fragments and chemotherapy or insulin pumps should not have MRIs.

Some people feel claustrophobic in the small MRI tube and this makes it difficult for them to lie quietly for the length of an MRI, which can last up to an hour for multiple scans

Cost (outside countries that have healthcare that covers MRIs) provides another barrier to obtaining an MRI. Many people either do not have insurance or face an expensive co-pay. Sometimes insurance carriers will deny coverage of an MRI, even for individuals with MS.

I find MRIs relaxing, but lying quietly and motionless on a metal table while MRI images are obtained with a great deal of noise can be difficult for some people. In addition, people with back pain or spasticity can find lying still on the hard table hard to do.

MRIs can also cause difficulty due to claustrophobia. For those with anxiety during an MRI, anti-anxiety medications may help. Learning to practice deep breathing, relaxation techniques, or meditation may increase one's tolerance of being in a small space. In addition, most MRI tables have a weight limit of 350 pounds. Anyone heavier cannot be imaged on typical MRI machines.

As for me, at 63 and having had MS for twenty years, I have had more MRIs than I can count. I've told my neurologist, "No more MRIs." When I mentioned this on an online MS support forum, some people begged to differ, and I understand why they disagreed with my decision. They are on MS medication and need the MRI to show their neurologists the state of their lesions. If their lesions have not diminished, the doctor may change the medication. In addition, if you have MS and you suddenly start to have issues, eye issues for instance, an MRI can show if you have developed lesions on your optic nerve. If you have, MS is most likely causing your eye problems. If you don't have lesions on your optic nerve, you should see an eye doctor.

In short, there are reasons for having MRIs, on an annual basis or once every couple of years. I would never suggest that anyone with MS should stop having them. All I am saying is that after 20 years of MRIs, I personally have had enough. And my neurologist, bless her heart, said she understood my decision.

11 / Living with MS

MS can sap your energy and cause a variety of debilitating physical sensations. But for many MS Warriors the disease doesn't have to stop you from living your life and doing what you want to do, more or less. You just have to work harder than most people to accomplish what you want, especially when you are having a relapse. Those with SPMS or PPMS will have to work even harder, but I know people with both of those types of MS, and they live lives that are quite inspirational, even those who are in wheelchairs.

With that in mind, here are some thoughts to help you live with MS. For what it's worth, I am not saying it's going to be easy. I am saying it's something worth working at.

Since energy levels often ebb and flow, try to schedule your days according to what you know about your energy levels. If you always get tired in the afternoon, try to get as much done as you can in the morning and vice versa. I know I'm not good for much of anything in the evenings, so I walk my dog in the mornings when my wife is busy and in the afternoons before it's time to crash on the couch. I write or I teach my online writing courses late mornings and early afternoons.

If you have a regular job, see if you can change your work schedule to get to the office early so you can leave before you're too tired. Do important jobs first and see if you can chunk big tasks into smaller ones that are more manageable.

Schedule regular breaks to restore your energy. If work can accommodate you, try to take a few 10- to 15-minute power naps during the day. If you work from home, as I do, nap as may be required and as your schedule allows. At the same time, don't nap too much. It could throw off your sleep schedule and keep you up at night. Rather than nap, I try to relax by reading a book or playing Words with Friends (the online Scrabble-type game). After dinner, I'll watch TV shows, mostly British dramas, that keep me engaged.

You do have to sleep. Unfortunately, sleep, hence rest, can be difficult for some people with MS. For instance, pain and muscle spasms can keep you up at night. Some of the medicines that treat MS interrupt sleep, too. Work with your doctor to get your medications under control so you can sleep. At the same time, if you are having difficulty sleeping, try reading. I find it helps me fall asleep or get back to sleep when I wake up in the middle of the night. In addition, Google "techniques to help you fall asleep." There are many other suggestions, beyond medications, online. Find something that works for you so you don't have to become drug-dependant to get a decent night's sleep.

For instance, avoid caffeine and alcohol within four to six hours of bedtime. Don't smoke before you go to sleep. Or better still, don't smoke at all (more on this later).

If running to the bathroom is keeping you awake, drink less in the evenings. Get your recommended amount of fluids during the day and use the restroom before you go to bed.

Stay active. You might not feel like getting up in the morning or you might feel like crawling between the covers during the day for a long nap, but try to keep moving. Our dog needs to be walked at least twice a day. He gets me out of the house, often for up to two hours. (He plays with other dogs in the park; I mostly sit on a bench and watch him, I confess.) But even a short walk will do to help you stay active.

You might also want to try some yoga or light exercise to keep yourself active.

Stay as cool as you can, unless cool temperatures bother you. For many with MS, heat and humidity can bring on fatigue or flares. That happened to me when I first developed MS. I couldn't take a hot shower or my MS tingles and my fatigue would grow more intense. If you start to lag when the temperature rises, stay inside where it's air-conditioned. Or try wearing a cooling vest. The most common type has insulated pockets that hold small ice packs. You wear it over your clothing, and it keeps you cool for several hours. You can also wear headbands or neckbands that use the same cooling methods.

Eat for energy not just for food fulfilment. Three big meals a day can drag you down, especially if they're heavy on fat, sugar, and carbohydrates. Instead, eat several smaller meals throughout the day. Eat meals that are nutrition rich. But more on diet and exercise later.

If your MS issues are cognitive, use tools to help you remember. For instance, carry a digital recorder. When you need to remember a name, phone number, or date, record a note to yourself. Write down the information or enter it into your computer when you get home.

I don't have MS-related cognitive issues, at least I have not been diagnosed with any, but I easily forget things. I will sometimes call my home phone from my cell phone and leave myself a message. Many people only have cell phones. If that is the case, send yourself a text or an email to help you remember important things. You can also use your cell phone camera to snap photos of new people, places, and things. Email pictures that you take to yourself with a note so you'll remember them later.

I have been using the calendar and task manager in Outlook, my email reader, since before I was diagnosed with MS. Every morning when I turn on my computer and open Outlook, the program reminds me of what I want to do. Your computer, cell phone or tablet should have calendar programs that can help you keep track of your schedule. But heck, you don't have to be a big fan of technology to assist your memory. Simply write important dates on an old-fashioned paper calendar. And carry a pad of paper and a pen with you so you can jot down notes as you go through your day.

You can also put a white board on your fridge or other area where you spend a lot of time. Write notes and to-do lists on it. Post-it notes are also a good way to jog your memory. Stick them around your house, office or in your car—places you know you will be so that you know you will see them.

Set up a box or bin by your front door for everyday items—keys, wallet, glasses and so on. You can also set aside a folder for important papers.

Driving and MS

People with MS often wonder if they should give up driving. I have stopped driving. If I got behind the wheel I would be like a drunk getting behind the wheel. My doctor did not tell me to stop driving. Common sense did.

For many with MS, to drive or not can be a difficult decision to make. Not driving can result in isolation and the need to rely on help from others. But if your disabilities are such that your reflexes or reaction times are at all impaired, giving up driving is something that you should seriously consider. If it helps, talk about this issue with your doctor. And if you can still safely drive with your MS, cool. Drive on!

Disability Benefits and MS

MS is such a chronic condition that having MS may force you to leave your job. If that is the case, you may qualify for disability benefits. The process to apply for disability can be long and frustrating. A lot may depend on the nature of laws where you live, the policies of the company your work for or on any insurance policies you or the company you work for have. If you are thinking of applying for disability, make sure you have your doctor(s) on board, and take a deep breath as you prepare for what may be a long and complex process.

12 / Life Hacks and MS

The term hacking is primarily used by computer experts who look for ways to create short cuts that will accelerate their workflow. However, a life hack refers to any trick, shortcut, skill, or method that increases personal productivity or that enables you to manage time and daily activities in a more efficient manner.

Living with MS can be challenging, but some simple lifestyle changes or hacks can help you overcome or better deal with many issues as your MS symptoms ebb and flow.

If you find running errands strenuous, for instance, consider using grocery-delivery services to deliver your goods or, if possible, order what you need in advance and simply pick up your order instead of walking around the store shopping for a list of goods.

If tired or fatigued, try taking power naps for 15 minutes or so, or if really fatigued, for an hour or so. Power naps can help you recharge your energy before an important event.

If you have gait and balance issues, consider using a cane, walker, scooter or wheelchair. These mobility assistive devices can make the difference between being housebound and getting around. Walkers with seats are great because you don't need to look for a chair if you need to sit and rest. If you can walk, but are easily fatigued, scoot to where you have to go, walk around to do what you have to do and then scoot home.

About 50 percent of people with MS will develop problems with cognition, according to the National Multiple Sclerosis Society. Brain-training apps and memory challenges can help you stay sharp. Try Sudoku (you can buy a puzzle book or download the app) or play Words with Friends (the Scrabble-type app). Many cognitive games can be loaded on your smart phone, tablet or computer and they can be a good way to exercise your brain.

Being forgetful can be a day-to-day struggle for some people with MS. If you are forgetful, make lists on paper or on portable computing devices that you can carry around with you. Don't forget to set reminders on your to-do list items so that your computing device reminds you about what you want to do and when you want to do it.

As mentioned in this book, many people with MS experience strange symptoms when they get overheated, whether from hot temperatures or during exercise. This can also occur when you have a fever. To help stay cool, drink cold water to cool off from the inside out. Also, put a cooling towel behind your neck. You can also buy or make cooling packs. To make yourself a cooling pack, combine three cups of water with one cup of rubbing alcohol in a re-sealable plastic bag and stick it in the freezer. The mixture gets freezing cold but doesn't freeze solid, resulting in a slush that stays cold for a couple of hours. There are also cooling towels you can wrap around yourself or cooling vests that you can wear on hot days or if you are exerting yourself and heating up at the gym.

Many people with MS experience bladder control problems like a frequent or urgent need to urinate. The best thing you can do if you are going to be away from home is scout out the bathrooms as soon as you arrive at your destination. You can also wear adult incontinence control devices to help you make it through the day if you are going to be out and about and not close to washrooms.

If you have dexterity issues, consider using dexterity kits to help you grip toothbrushes, door knobs, utensils, pens and other items you need to hold on to. You can also get zipper pulls, which are so much easier than trying to maneuver small zipper tabs. Magnetic button-down shirts, originally developed for Parkinson's patients, look like regular shirts, but the buttons are actually magnets that require almost zero fine motor skills.

When it comes to taking showers, we have installed bars in our shower that I can hold on to while I am under the shower spray and we have a stool I can sit on so that I can wash my legs and feet. Also consider using a walk-in tub. Getting one could mean an expensive bathroom modification but it is great for avoiding a fall while trying to step in and out of the bathtub.

There are hacks to help you overcome most, but not all, issues. Do a quick Google search to find the most current ones that are out there. They won't cure your MS or defeat your symptoms, but they might make life a bit easier for you to cope with.

Having said that, I know it's easy to feel down or blue when you have MS, even if you are using life hacks to assist you. With that in mind, the book includes a chapter on doing your best to deal with depression.

13 / MS and Exercise

Research has shown that there are benefits associated with increased physical activity for those with MS—as long as your body lets you exercise. An American study published in 1996 helped shift the thinking about MS and exercise. The study examined the effects of fifteen weeks of aerobic exercise in people with MS compared to those who did no exercise. The study found that those who participated in the exercise program experienced reduced fatigue, depression and anger and improved their overall quality of life. So if you can exercise—walk, jog, cycle, pump iron, and so on—you should do so as it will help improve your aerobic endurance, muscular strength, flexibility, overall mobility and state of mind.

I get to walk our dog every day, rain, snow or shine. There are days when I really don't want to walk, and then ten minutes into the walk I'm glad that I'm out there, even if my legs are stiff as they usually are. I used to ride my bike in all seasons but winter for at least an hour a day. I had to give up biking about twelve years ago because MS has weakened my legs. But at least I can still walk the dog.

In some instances, exercise can help ease your MS symptoms, but you have to be careful when you workout. The most important thing is this: Don't overdo it. You know the saying "no pain, no gain"? Well, when you have MS you don't need pain to gain. In fact, doing too much can strain your muscles, put too much stress on your body and exacerbate fatigue or any MS pain or other symptoms that you have. However, proper exercise can keep your muscles flexible and strong.

Not all people with MS can exercise. Many can only exercise in a limited manner. Some can get in a light workout and some can work out quite vigorously, especially if they have RRMS and are in remission.

If you are fatigued, if you can barely walk, if you need assistance moving (use a cane, walker or a wheelchair) exercise may be the last thing on your mind. You might even want to skip this chapter. I would not blame you. But I am going to ask you to read it, to read about the importance of exercise to our physical and mental well being. I am going to ask you to dig as deep as you can and do whatever you are capable of doing to keep yourself as fit as possible.

Some of us might be able to do a fair bit. Others might not be able to do much at all. In either case, allow me to say this: there is no shame in limitations. Do what you can do, knowing that what you can do is good for you. It's good for both your physical and mental well being.

Exercise gives you more energy during the day and helps you sleep better at night. Regular physical activity also improves your balance. At the same time, don't exercise to the point of exhaustion as it tends to take those with MS longer to recover from a vigorous workout, or even a mild one.

You can exercises alone, or you can work with a physical therapist who can help you build a personal exercise program that meets your needs and can show you how to do each exercise movement safely and effectively. Whatever you do, check with your doctor before you start any fitness program. Talk to your doctor about the types of exercise that are best for you and those you should avoid, about how long and intense your workouts should be and about any physical limitations you should keep in mind.

With professional advice in mind, you might want to try aerobics to get your heartbeat up and help lift your mood. Walking, running, and biking are all good. If you have leg weakness or other problems moving, try something like rowing or water aerobics.

As mentioned, stretches are good for anyone with MS. They are most helpful if you have painful muscle stiffness and spasms. Aside from regular stretches, yoga and tai chi are great ways to build strength and flexibility. They can also help you relax and fight stress.

If you have RRMS and go into remission, continue to exercise. You want your body to be as strong as possible to help you deal with any potential relapses. If you relapse, you may have to pull back on the amount of exercise you do, but continue to do what you can do to stay in the best possible shape.

Tips for a Safe Workout

It's a good idea to combine three types of exercise:

Strength training. To keep your muscles strong, work them with light weights or exercise bands a couple of times a week. If you get a muscle spasm in the middle of your routine, stop and wait a few minutes for it to relax. Also, stop if you feel any pain. Exercise should never hurt.

Range of motion. To prevent stiffness, do exercises that take your joints through their full range of motion. For example, lift your arm up and over your head, or bring your leg out to the side and back.

Stretching. Do a series of stretches at least twice a week, if not once a day. Pay special attention to muscles that tend to get tight and spasm, like the quadriceps, hamstrings, and calves. As you stretch out each muscle, hold the stretch for up to one minute and then gently release it.

When you are working out, keep the tips below in mind.

Always warm up with some light stretches before you start your exercise routine. Ease into your routine rather than sprint into it.

Work on stretches and strength training to improve your balance and coordination.

If all you can do is a walk around the block, or across the room, that's fine. Start with that and keep it up. In time, the hope is that you will build up your strength and be able to do more.

To stay safe, avoid places with slippery floors, poor lighting, throw rugs, or other tripping hazards. You may want to have a grab bar or rail nearby when you are working out. On the other hand, you can choose activities that will eliminate the chance of a fall, like stationary biking or swimming.

As I said, I walk the dog at least once a day. He gets me outside and moving. (He is also a great indoor companion!) See if you can find ways to motivate yourself to exercise regularly.

14 / MS and Diet

Can diet help alleviate your MS?

Pretend for a moment that you don't have MS. If you eat poorly, you will feel poor. If you eat well, you will feel pretty good. But you have MS. So if you eat poorly, you will feel poor on top of any MS symptoms you are experiencing. If you eat well, you will feel as best you can on top of any symptoms. And your good diet just might help you keep your MS symptoms at bay or at least help to minimize them.

Most doctors recommend you eat a low-fat, high-fiber diet similar to the one recommended for the general public by major medical organizations. They also suggest you take daily doses of vitamin D. Some suggest vitamin B-12 as well. Again, these are not cures. These are ways to keep you feeling as well as you can feel while, hopefully, combating your flare ups and symptoms.

When first diagnosed with MS there was one thing that I did with my diet that helped me with my overall energy. I found a book called *Fit For Life* by Harvey and Marilyn Diamond. I think I ate pretty well before following the *Fit For Life* diet. But I did have a bit of a junk food streak in me.

The basic premise of the *Fit for Life* book is this: fruit, and only fruit, for breakfast, and no mixing carbohydrates (breads, potatoes, rice and other starches) with protein (chicken, fish, beef and other meat). In other words, you can't be a meat and potatoes guy on this diet.

You know how at Thanksgiving you have a heaping helping of turkey, mashed potatoes and a sugary dessert, and then basically pass out? Well that's the antithesis of the fit for life diet. Have that turkey with a salad and guess what? You have energy to burn. So while following the diet did not get rid of my MS symptoms, including fatigue, it did seem to lessen my fatigue and boost my energy in between bouts of fatigue.

Am I saying your should follow the diet? Not at all. But if energy, or lack thereof, is your issue, it can't hurt to try it for a couple of months to see what happens to your energy levels.

People with MS sometimes wonder if they should go gluten free. Doing so can't hurt you but no research has shown that a gluten free diets improve MS symptoms. If you are at all curious, try it for a few months and see how you feel. If you feel better, carry on. If you feel the same, or worse, stop avoiding gluten.

The Palaeolithic (Paleo) diet has been in the news a fair bit recently. Paleo diets favor lean meats, nuts, and berries. The Paleo approach stems from the idea that your body can process these ancient staples better than modern items, such as dairy products and processed carbohydrates. In one small study, people with MS who followed the Paleo diet for a year said they were less tired than people who didn't. But that might not just be about their diet, since the people on the Paleo diet also exercised, stretched, and meditated during the study.

Still, it can't hurt you to try the diet if you are experimenting with the impact that food has on your MS. Same with the Mediterranean diet, a diet in which you eat a lot of fish, whole grains, fruits and vegetables, legumes, and olive oil. There's no research on how this diet affects MS in particular. But many studies show that it's good for you overall and may help lower inflammation.

A couple of people that I know who have MS have tossed all their medications and are now on the Wahls Protocol diet. The diet is a version of the Paleo diet. It's based on the idea that humans should eat more like our ancient ancestors ate and avoid the foods we started eating in the past several hundred years, like wheat and processed foods.

On the Wahls Protocol, you eat a lot of meat and fish, vegetables (especially green, leafy ones), brightly colored fruit (like berries), fat from animals and plant sources, especially omega-3 fatty acids. But you don't eat dairy products and eggs, grains (including wheat, rice, and oatmeal), legumes (beans and lentils), nightshade vegetables (tomatoes, eggplant, potatoes and peppers) or sugar.

So does the Wahls Protocol work for people with MS? Wahls, who was diagnosed with MS, says her diet helped her go from using a wheelchair to biking for miles. While her personal experience may sound promising, there isn't a lot of research yet that shows that the diet works for others with MS. However, one small study found that people with MS who switched to a Wahls-style diet for a year were less tired. But those people also exercised and did stretches, meditated and got massage therapy and electrical stimulation therapy. So it's hard to say that the diet alone helped them with their symptoms.

In other words, the jury is still out, but other studies are taking place. Again though, it doesn't seem like the diet can hurt you. There is a lot of information about the diet online. To start with, you can visit the Wahls' website, terrywahls.com. In addition, Wahls has written several books about the diet, one being *The Wahls Protocol: How I Beat Progressive MS Using Paleo Principles and Functional Medicine*. Google Terry Wahls at any online bookstore to see her books.

As always, talk to your doctor before starting any particular diet.

Foods to Avoid

Saturated fats come primarily from animal products and by-products such as red meat and dairy. They're also in foods that contain palm oil and coconut oil. Saturated fats are known to raise your LDL, or bad cholesterol, which can cause heart problems. According to studies, people who have MS are at an increased risk for heart problems. In addition, hypertension and cardiovascular disease are thought to make MS worse. So you might want to think seriously about avoiding saturated fats.

You should also skip foods with trans fats, like commercially baked cookies, crackers, pies, and any other packaged products. Key words to look for on nutrition labels to identify such products are "partially hydrogenated oils" and "shortening."

Too much sugar, especially in the form of sweets, can cause weight gain and you don't want to increase your weight as that can make it more difficult for you to be mobile. Excess weight also increases fatigue. In addition, sugar is an inflammatory food that may have a negative effect on your symptoms.

Beware of too much sodium or salt. A study found that the more sodium in the diets of people who have MS, the more likely they were to relapse, and the greater their risk of developing new lesions.

Watch out for white foods such as white rice, white bread and cold breakfast cereals. These processed carbohydrates can elevate blood sugar levels and negatively affect your heart health. Consider switching to whole-grain bread, brown rice, barley and whole-wheat pasta. These high-fiber options are better overall for you and they can help you manage constipation, an MS symptom for some.

In summary, eat a variety of fruits and vegetables, whole grains, low-fat dairy products, skinless poultry and fish, nuts and legumes. Avoid items that are highly processed and high in saturated fat. In other words, eat your vegetables and avoid junk food, as best you can.

MS and Vitamins

Although no vitamin supplement can cure MS, some vitamin therapies can help reduce symptoms or prolong periods of remission. However, just as the disease is different for everyone who has it, so is the reaction to vitamins for those with MS.

Vitamin D is one of the most studied supplements for MS. It seems as if low vitamin D levels may lead to an increased risk of MS exacerbations. Daily supplements up to 4,000 international units (IU) of vitamin D-3 is generally considered safe. Doses greater than 4,000 IU a day may be necessary in people who are vitamin D deficient, but large doses may also carry increased risks. Because people absorb vitamin D differently, talk to your doctor to determine if checking your blood levels could help identify the right dose for you.

According to the MS Society of Canada, a growing body of evidence demonstrates that vitamin D deficiency is associated with MS. Studies have shown that the risk of developing MS is decreased with either higher levels of vitamin D intake. While the association between vitamin D status and MS risk is quite strong, it is less clear whether vitamin D supplements can improve disease outcomes in people living with MS. Clinical trials are currently evaluating the role of vitamin D in altering the disease course.

Vitamins B6 and B12, which play an important role in the functioning of our nervous systems by helping to maintain the myelin sheath, may also assist those with MS.

Alcohol and MS

Can you drink alcohol if you have MS? That is a question people with MS ask.

I don't drink alcohol any more. That's because my chronic headaches and leg issues make me feel somewhat unstable. I don't need alcohol to add to my instability. Some people with MS assert that the occasional drink helps them get through the day.

According to various studies, alcohol has a number of short-term effects that can exacerbate many of the symptoms of MS. On the other hand, there have been studies that suggest a couple of glasses of wine per week might help ease symptoms.

What you don't want to do is abuse alcohol as that can exacerbate your symptoms, not to mention that alcohol abuse could also damage the liver, stomach, and other organs. Just what you don't need if you have MS.

The effects of alcohol on those with MS may just depend upon the type of MS one has. For instance, alcohol in moderation may be less harmful to those with RRMS than to those with PPMS. Of course how people with MS react to alcohol will vary, as everything seems to be different for everybody with MS.

By way of aside, people with MS also wonder if they can drink coffee. While there is no association between coffee and the exacerbation of symptoms, if you have bladder problems coffee could make them worse. So coffee may not have a detrimental effect on your MS, but it could have a negative impact on your symptoms.

Smoking and MS

While smoking isn't part of your diet, you do ingest smoke and all the tar, nicotine and other chemicals in cigarettes, so let's pretend it's a food.

Smokers have higher rates of lung cancer, heart disease, emphysema and other respiratory problems. Smoking also produces shortness of breath, susceptibility to lung infections and heartbeat irregularities. These irregularities might transform neurological issues in a person with MS into more severe symptoms. In addition, smoking may actually increase the risk of developing MS.

According to a Norwegian study, the risk of MS was significantly higher among smokers than among those who had never smoked. Doesn't mean non-smokers won't get MS; just means smokers seem to be more susceptible to it.

Another study supported evidence that smoking is a risk factor in the development and progression of MS. The study in the journal *Brain* supported the link between smoking and the risk of developing MS and suggested that smoking may transform RRMS into a SPMS. Researchers reported links between smoking and lesions observed on MRI scans of people with MS.

So if you have MS, or even don't have it, you now have another reason to butt out.

15 / MS and Depression

People with MS often get depressed, just like people without it get depressed. Depression is different for everyone, but coupled with a debilitating disease it can be incredibly crippling.

For instance, if you have PPMS and your legs are going, or perhaps gone, and you need a wheel chair to move around, that's depressing. Perhaps you have SPMS and your symptoms will not abate, that's depressing. Perhaps you have RRMS and your are having a flare that keeps you from working and interferes with your interactions with others. That can get you down

When I was first diagnosed with MS, I freaked out. I was not an MS Warrior then. I had a wife and seven-year-old daughter and no life insurance, and I thought I was going to die. I'm sure the neurologist explained that I wasn't going to drop dead, but it felt like I had just been handed a death sentence. So I had to learn how to adjust my attitude as I was learning how to cope with my MS

I am not saying you should be depressed if you have MS. I know people with MS who maintain a positive and upbeat attitude. I am saying, though, that if you have MS I certainly would not blame for feeling down or blue because of your condition. The fact is, we sometimes have to fight hard to feel good about ourselves and our lives, given our condition. And fight we should, especially given our condition.

The fact is, it's bad enough that you are sick. Try your best to not be down about it too—other than those occasional moments when you allow yourself to crawl into a corner and scream to high heaven about the unfairness of it all. I will allow you those moments if you promise me that you will wipe away the tears and bounce back and laugh about it all, even though it is not funny. Deal? Deal

But if I may back up for a moment, I want to say this about depression: if you are experiencing deep depression, or what is known as clinical depression, you should talk to your doctor because you may need some kind of talk therapy to help you overcome that kind of depression. However, if you are coping with life overall but feeling blue about your life with MS, there are some things you can do to help you combat the blues.

What I try to do to combat depression is to distract myself from my blue moods. Writing this book helps. I also participate in several MS support forums on Facebook and I belong to an in-person support group. In addition, I blog a bit, watch good movies and television shows, read books and play Words with Friends and Yahtzee with Buddies on my tablet. With that in mind, consider taking up a hobby: music, painting, writing (start a blog, for instance), knitting, weaving, woodworking, dollhouse making, ceramics, pottery, collecting, designing… Anything that keeps you engaged and mentally active and, as I said, distracted from what you are going through and dealing with.

In addition, regular exercise can also help you beat the blues by boosting levels of the brain's natural feel-good chemicals. For instance, a pet, as long as you can care for it, can be a source of comfort. Our dog needs to be walked twice a day and so he gets me out of the house and into fresh air. Often I walk him to the nearby dog park and sit on a bench and watch him play. While I may not be getting a whole lot of exercise, I get to sit on a park bench and talk to other dog owners and almost feel normal.

How to Anticipate and Relieve Stress

Stress can trigger and worsen MS symptoms. This is ironic in that once you are diagnosed with MS there is a very good chance that you will feel stressed. To help manage your emotions, it helps to learn the warning signs that indicate that stress is headed your way.

When stress is about to hit, your body sends out physical, emotional, and behavioral warning signs. Try to be in tune with these signs. Some of the emotional signals you may notice are that you get angry easily, find it hard to concentrate, feel perpetually worried or sad or have frequent mood swings.

There are physical warning signs too. They include stooped posture, sweaty palms or weight gain or loss. In addition, you might find yourself overreacting, acting on impulse, using alcohol or drugs or withdrawing from relationships.

So what can you do to reduce stress, once you acknowledge that you are feeling stressed out?

Part of your strategy to reduce stress is to keep a positive attitude and accept that there are some events that you are not able to control. I know, easier said than done, so you may have to dig deep to keep your attitude as positive as possible.

In addition, try to follow these stress reduction tips:

Express your feelings, instead of holding them in and becoming angry, combative or extremely passive.

Learn and use relaxation techniques, such as yoga, meditation, deep breathing or muscle and mind relaxation techniques, to help yourself stay calm.

Listen to and relax to soothing music and let go of as much tension as you can.

Find a distraction to engage you, ideally something you are passionate about.

Exercise regularly to the extent you can.

Eat well-balanced meals.

Get enough rest and sleep.

In short, don't rely on alcohol or drugs to reduce stress. All they will do is leave you feeling even bluer, especially when you come down from your artificial high. Try to engage your body and your mind. Again, try to find a distraction or engage in something that you are interested in or about which you are passionate. That might help and it beats the alternative: sitting on the couch or in your wheelchair feeling sorry for yourself.

Again, I am not saying you should never feel down or even angry about MS. I am saying you shouldn't stay down or that anger should not be your prominent emotion.

In addition to stress, fatigue is a common symptom of MS. If you're not getting enough sleep, this can have a negative impact on your energy and emotional levels. So try to get six to eight hours of sleep a night and rest during the day if your body needs it.

To help you sleep better, try relaxation techniques like meditation, yoga, or deep breathing before you go to bed. Reading while in bed can also help. I have a Kobo Glo electronic reader (e-reader) that is backlit and lets me read in the dark so I don't have to turn on lights to read (there is a Kindle e-reader that is also backlit).

Things to Avoid

There are things that those of us with MS should try exceptionally hard not to do, no matter our condition.

For instance, we should not sit around feeling sorry for ourselves. No matter how bad you have it somebody else has it worse. Knowing that isn't going to cure you of your MS and it may not even make you feel any better, knowing that it could be worse. I guess what I am trying to say is that you should try to keep what you are going through, as much as it sucks, in perspective.

That others have it worse, I want to stress, should not make you feel any better in the least. It doesn't help me. But my hope is that it will help you keep your life in perspective, and that perspective will help you fight hard to overcome your blue feelings.

We should not lash out, at ourselves or at others. After all, where does lashing out get you? MS is arbitrary and unfair. We know that. Many things in life are arbitrary and unfair. But MS is not our fault and it is not the fault of anybody around us.

Nobody, if I may editorialize here for a moment, deserves to be the victim of vitriol and anger. Those of us with MS don't deserve it, from ourselves or from those around us who may have difficulty coping with our condition. And those around us don't deserve it because we are having difficulty accepting and coping with our condition.

Having said that, I sure as hell don't blame anybody for feeling blue or down. I get blue, down and depressed at times. In fact, writing about how you should try your best to stay positive and upbeat has me, at this moment, feeling kind of down. But I will bounce back because I don't like wallowing in the gutter. I sure as hell don't like my MS, but I like it all even less when I am feeling down about it.

So try as best you can to put in place a program, a life it's called, that keeps you mentally and physically active and keeps you out of the dumps, or at least keeps you a much lighter shade of blue as you deal with MS and all it entails.

16 / Communicating about MS

MS, unless you are in a wheelchair or are using a walker, is a hidden disease. If you look at me you can't see my headaches or my leg weakness. If someone has severe brain fog, you can't see his or her brain in a cluttered mess. If someone has shooting pains in their jaw, legs, chest or joints, how can you see that? You might know that a person has MS but you also might forget because the person looks fine. You simply can't see what's going on in her or his body. But there is stuff going on, as you have seen from the information in this book.

Once you learn you have MS, it may take you some time to adjust to your symptoms and to know what to expect from your disease. The most important thing to do, once you get a fix on what you are going through, is to talk to people in your life—family members, friends, work associates, and so on—about how MS affects you. Open communication can give those close to you a chance to ask questions and ease any particular fears or concerns that they may have.

I am not saying it will be easy to talk about your MS. I am not saying that everyone you talk to will be accepting and understanding. In fact, some people won't accept and understand. Some people might even desert you. But what is the alternative? To suffer in silence? To have flare ups and to try to keep them hidden? I am saying that talking to others, as difficult as it may be, is something you should try to do.

The sad fact is MS can take a toll on your relationships. If your symptoms flare, you might not be able to go to family dinners or social events. You may feel that you've let people down. You haven't; you are sick and can't help how you feel. At the same time, the people around you might feel like you have let them down. You haven't; you are sick. But you need to deal with your feelings and those of the people around you, as best you can.

I know that dealing with MS has caused couples to break up and friends and even family members to desert those who are ill. In a moment of frustration, one husband whose wife has MS yelled at her, "I didn't ask for this." Two points. One: neither did your wife. Two: technically, you did: 'In sickness and in health.' But the fact is that MS, or any chronic illness, can put a strain on your relationships. You might be less independent and need to rely on your partner for care at times, like helping you bathe or driving you to doctor's appointments. This can be stressful—for both of you.

Make sure your spouse knows that you appreciate their support and love. Talk about financial concerns and other stress factors. If your partner feels they do more than their share, let them know you're aware of that. Find solutions to problems together or get counselling if you need it.

I am not saying that relationship difficulties will occur. I am saying they have occurred with many couples who have had to deal with MS. At the same time, dealing with MS has brought some families and friends closer together as the people around the MS Warrior help him or her cope with the disease.

What I am suggesting here is that people have to talk things through and determine how to handle various scenarios. I am not suggesting that such conversations will be easy; they may even be painful. But they are necessary.

The fact is, the result of conversations may be that a couple decides to split up, but at least they have talked it over and, I hope, reached an amicable decision that both parties have agreed to—in other words, they know what they are doing and why they are doing it. In short, all you can do is be open and honest and hope those around you are understanding and accepting.

And if your partner has MS, keep in mind that there are things you can avoid saying. The online MS support group, myMSteam.com, has listed some of the worst advice friends and family members have given people with MS. Comments include the following statements:

You should get out more
Just push through it
You don't look disabled
Everyone gets tired sometimes
Have you tried vitamins?
You should go back to work
But you look fine
Just move around more

Pretty lame stuff, I think you would agree.

I don't know how else to put it. Listen to your ill partner or ill friend. Hear what they have to say. Take them seriously. Acknowledge what they have to say. Sympathize with them. Don't tell them you know how they feel; you don't.

Don't give them unsolicited advice. But let them know you are there for them. Find out what they would like to do, and then give them some of your time and do it—even if it is just sitting there for a bit doing nothing, saying next to nothing. Do that because understanding and empathy is about all you can give someone with MS. It may not sound like much, but it means one heck of a lot to the person with MS, or to someone with any chronic illness.

Talking to Children

If you have children, before you sit down to talk to them, think about their age, maturity level, and how much you think they can understand about your disease. If you have more than one child, it may be helpful to talk to them individually so you can tailor the discussion to each child.

You may want to ask your children how they would like to learn more about MS. They can start by reading a book or online information alone or with you, watching an online video or going with you to a doctor's visit. Don't be surprised if your kids already know that something is up before you talk about it with them. Children of all ages are good at knowing when things are different.

Sometimes normal emotions like fear, sadness or guilt may lead to changes in a child's behaviour. Watch how your children react, pay attention to their behaviour. Continue to talk to them and, if necessary, get some professional assistance in communicating with them.

In summary, let the people close to you know how MS affects your body and mind. Talk with friends or family about what's going on with your health. Tell them why you may have to skip some activities.

But don't look at yourself as a person with an illness. You're much more than your MS. Keep a positive self-image and work on maintaining positive relationships. And if someone deserts you because they are unable to cope with the changes in your life that MS may necessitate, be the bigger person and learn how to let them go.

17 / Healthy Partners of MS Warriors

MS hurts people who have it, often dramatically changing their lives. They may have to quit work. They may have less quality time to spend with family and friends. They may be frequently fatigued. I could go on but at this point in the book you get the picture.

At the same time, MS can hurt partners of those who have it. They may have to pick up the burden of taking care of things that their partners used to take care of. They may feel deserted, alone and even exhausted by the extra work that they have to do, from the care they are providing and from the constant concern.

Let's face it, care giving is a challenging, one that can increase bonds between people and one that can also destroy relationships. That is why I wanted to let healthy partners of MS Warriors speak. I offered them anonymity so that they would feel free to speak their minds. And so the next words you read belong to healthy partners of those with MS.

* * *

Amongst the people I know who have MS, I've known several that have had their loved ones stay by their side. I've known just as many who've had their relationships fall apart. Whether it's the lack of information or the fear of looking down the uncertain road ahead, I'm not sure. Maybe it's just a convenient excuse to end a relationship. I know that I found the uncertainty difficult to take.

We just couldn't do what we used to do together and my wife just seemed to be getting sicker and sicker. So, sadly, we split up. She is with family now and I support her financially, but there just wasn't a solid relationship to hold together any longer.

* * *

I am currently in a relationship with someone who has MS. There are good days and they there are difficult days. Sometimes the good days go on for weeks or months and sometimes the difficult ones go on just as long. We love each other so we are battling through the bad times together. I really don't know what else to say. I am being as supportive as I can be but I also know my partner has a lot to deal with, physically and emotionally. I just have to deal with it emotionally.

Our future is something that is uncertain, that we know. But day to day, we are more or less doing okay. I'm not saying it's easy for me, but compared to what she is going through, I guess I have it easy. It just doesn't feel that way because MS has changed our relationship and what we can and cannot do together and what she can and cannot do. And I have to pick up the slack.

I work fulltime and we don't have children. For that I am grateful. Although doctors tell us we could have kids, we have decided that we don't want to bring children into this equation.

* * *

My partner has had RRMS for about a decade. There have been good times and a lot of bad times when he has been fatigued or had mobility issues.

When he was first diagnosed we knew nothing about this disease. We got some information from his neurologist and we got a lot of information about MS online. Still, it seems like such a strange disease in the way it manifest itself. We didn't know what would happen.

When he was first diagnosed, my partner was very depressed and I felt helpless. As his symptoms abated his sprits picked up and life returned to normal, more of less. But MS symptoms keep on coming back. I guess we are more used to the strange issues he has to deal with. He is less depressed about his fatigue and mobility issues and I do more around the house. He works from home but has had to cut back on the work he does. That has hit our income, but we've made financial adjustments and I continue to work, which is not a problem. Although I have much more to do around the house and I get tired. I'm not comparing my getting tired to his fatigue, but there are times I could sure use a good, long break from what we are dealing with.

We have had a number of long talks. We are committed to each other and will continue to play the hand we've been dealt. It doesn't mean we like it; it means we are dealing with it as best we can.

* * *

My husband was diagnosed with PPMS about 15 years ago. It's been gut-wrenchingly sad to watch him go from walking, to using a cane, to using a scooter to needing a wheelchair to get around. I'm impressed by his overall attitude, as are our two kids. They are both in college now and living their lives, which we encourage them to do.

Some days I think my husband is dealing with his MS better than I am, even though he had to leave his job and go on long-term disability. It's been a challenge for us, but we've adjusted as best we can.

We had ramps put up to the doors so he can get in and out of the house. He basically lives on the first floor now. I have a pottery studio in the basement. At first when I'd go down there I'd feel like I was deserting him. But he pointed out that I used to go down there when he was well, and he wouldn't follow me down. So I continue to do my pottery.

We don't go out like we used to, but he has encouraged me to go out with friends and we still have friends over. Sometimes after dinner we'll watch a movie with our friends and he will fall asleep, but we've gotten used to it. It's as if he's slipping away, little by little. And he knows this. But as he says, he could have had a heart attack and dropped dead. He's still here, even if there is less of him here.

I think he's been very courageous in dealing with this disease, and that has somehow inspired me to become a better, more caring, person.

* * *

When my wife was diagnosed with MS our kids were five and seven. I think dealing with the children, explaining to them that "mom is sick" has been the most difficult things, beyond dealing with her symptoms, which are mostly fatigue and brain fog. The kids are older now, in their late teens, and they have learned to fend for themselves as my wife's symptoms have become more severe. There are days when about all she can do is move from the bed to the couch. I don't really know what to say. I'm still here. Maybe if we hadn't had kids the MS might have put an end to our relationship. But we had kids before she got sick and I am committed to being the best father and the best husband that I can be, under the circumstances. And my wife does what she can while dealing with this disease.

I read about some partners and family members who think the person with MS is just lazy or faking it. That gets me angry. I can only speak for my wife, but she was one of the most vital people I knew, before she became ill. She worked until we started our family. Then she was an active and involved caregiver and volunteered at our children's school. If anybody was a slob in this relationship, it was me! I've picked up the pace as best I can, and my kids are terrific. They understand that mom is sick and doing the best she can do. I guess if there is one thing that I'd want to say, this would be it: Do the best you can as you deal with the circumstances of MS. I mean, what more can you do?

*   *   *

MS is a pain in the butt to deal with. When my partner first got the diagnosis and was exhibiting all sort of symptoms—pain, tiredness, mobility issues—I confess I thought MS would be the end of us. She didn't want it and I didn't want to be a part of it. It took a while, but we started to talk about it and the implications of MS. Not sure who initiated the discussion, although I think she did. It was shortly after she started going to an MS support group in the area. I guess she learned how other couples were dealing with it. Some had broken up, she told me. But a lot of couples were doing okay.

Anyway, talking about it helped keep us together as we sorted out who would do what and I understood better what she was going through. And then, miracle of miracles, she started feeling better. I think we kind of went into denial about MS during that time, a couple of good years with just minor MS hits. But it's come back, not with a vengeance but the symptoms are bad enough that there is a lot of stuff that I now have to do. So I do it. Because that's what has to be done to keep our house in order and to keep ourselves together. I'm not saying that it's been easy, but we are making the best of a situation that we both wish were a lot better and easier to deal with.

*   *   *

Would it be selfish to say that sex, or a lack of it, has been an issue? I mean I understand that my wife is not in the mood because of her MS symptoms and depression. I'm sure if I were ill like she is I wouldn't be much in the mood either, although I'm a guy and guys are always in the mood. But overall, we are doing what we can do to deal with what MS has brought upon us.

Her energy is below par, so we don't go out like we used to. However, we order in and we got a new flat screen TV we can watch movies on. Also, she has taken up baking great desserts when she has the energy. So I guess in many ways great food has replaced sex. I mean I really do understand, as best I can, what she is going through. And she understands the impact it has had on me. Fact is nobody signs up for this so I'm not going to make her life any worse than it is, with her being sick and dealing with this incredibly stupid disease.

18 / Sex and Pregnancy

I want to say something brief about MS and sex here.

The human sex drive is complex. Emotional issues can have an impact on the sex drive. Physical issues can have an impact on one's sex drive too. MS can cause emotional and physical issues, as can any illnesses. In fact, you don't even need to be ill to have emotional or physical issues. I think it is called "life."

I am obviously not a sex therapist, so I don't really know what to say beyond the fact that MS can have a negative emotional and physical impact on your sex drive. If that happens, and for most people with MS it will, talk to your partner: see if you can replace sex with something else you can do together, such as cooking an incredible gourmet meal or going out for dinner and a movie or rubbing each others' feet.

Perhaps sit, cuddle and watch a couple episodes of The Great British Bake Off—the food is orgasmic! (And yes, like sex, the baking sometimes flops.) In other words, there is more to life than sex. Just snuggling up and being together in a warm, caring and loving manner can be a fulfilling part of your relationship.

In short, some people with MS are so disabled and/or distraught that any form of sexual activity is simply not possible. I am not saying give up on sex; I am saying it might not happen, or that it might not happen with the frequency and intensity of sex before MS. That doesn't mean you have to give up on intimacy!

Whatever you do, don't blame yourself (or your partner if your partner has MS). Nobody is responsible for MS or the impact it has on sexual appetite, or any appetite for that matter. I mean look at what MS did to my freaking taste buds, how it destroyed them for several months! Keep that in mind and live as well as you can live. Be patient. Be gentle. And be understanding. Nobody asked for this, but whoever has it has to live with it. If your partner has MS, don't make their life any more difficult than it is. And trust me, it is difficult—physically, mentally and emotionally. So be loving and caring. It's who your partner needs you to be. And you will become a better, stronger, more mature and more complete person for being that way.

I know we live in a sex-obsessed society. That doesn't mean you have to be obsessed with it. In fact, if you are not having sex, look at all the time you are saving and can apply to other, more meaningful, tasks. In short, if sex, or the lack of it, becomes an issue, take a deep breath and see what else you can do that is mutually fulfilling.

About Pregnancy

Far too many of those diagnosed with MS are young women. Many of them plan on having children. There is good news: if you want to start a family, having MS doesn't have to stop you. It doesn't keep you from getting pregnant or hurt your unborn baby. Odds are that your pregnancy and delivery will be just like a woman without MS.

In fact, according to studies, MS symptoms often stabilize or improve during pregnancies. Unfortunately though, about a third of women with MS who have a child have a relapse following delivery. However, the overall disease progression and the risk of additional relapses are not affected by pregnancy.

Still, moms-to-be with MS face unique challenges. With that in mind, new mothers should plan for more rest and assistance during pregnancy and after childbirth. It is recommended that you build a support team. Don't be afraid to ask family and friends to fix meals or help around the house so you can save your energy.

Before you try to get pregnant, talk to your doctor. Let her know you want to have a baby. If your MS is under control, you'll probably get a green light. If you are on medication and thinking of trying to get pregnant, your doctor may adjust your medication because some MS medications can increase the risk of miscarriage and may be transmitted in breast milk. In other words, you want to make sure that the medication you are taking to help you cope with your MS will not harm your child.

Once you are pregnant, be aware of urinary tract infections (UTIs). They are more common for pregnant women with MS. Drink lots of water, and tell your doctor if you feel burning when you go to the bathroom or if your urine is cloudy. You may get monthly urine tests to check for UTIs.

Pediatricians suggest that new mothers breastfeed for at least the first year of the life of their babies. That doesn't change because you have MS. You can't pass MS to your child through breast milk. And breast milk has the vitamins and nutrition your growing baby needs, as well as antibodies that boost their developing immune systems. A study found that breastfed babies of moms with MS were less likely than formula-fed babies to get ear infections and other typical newborn health problems during their first year.

So if you have MS and were planning to have a child, talk to your doctor. With a few adjustments, as may be required, you will most likely get the green light to go ahead and get pregnant.

19 / MS and Me

Currently, with my MS, I have chronic headaches 24/7. They are relentless. Plus I have some balance issues, weakness in my legs and some fatigue. Don't get me wrong. I am glad I can do what I can do. I know people with MS who are in better physical shape than I am, but they have brain fog or cognitive issues. Other people that I know with MS have to use walkers to get around. I use a cane, but can walk without it, although I appreciate the feeling of stability that it gives me. And still others with MS are confined to wheelchairs.

As said, my MS started with a strange tingling in my fingers. Over the day it spread into my hands. It was as if my fingers and hands were asleep. You know, that needles and pins sensation. I tried to shake it out, but the strange sensation remained. The next day it spread into my arms. And then up my arms into my chest and shoulders and down my back. It was as if my body was slowly falling asleep.

In short, I felt funny. Until it started to head south. Yes, my testicles started to tingle, and not in a good way. Then my legs and finally my feet succumbed to the strange sensations. At that point I told Lyn that I was experiencing a strange needles and pins sensation throughout my entire body. She was understandably concerned and suggested that I see my doctor. I wanted to give it a bit more time. After all, other than the strange sensation, I felt fine. And I'm a guy. We don't see doctors unless our heads are about to fall off, and only then if the duct tape has failed to keep it secure.

I kept on waiting for my body to wake up. But it wouldn't. And then the fatigue hit.

It wasn't all fatigue all the time. Nothing like that. I would be working—sitting at my computer writing an article—and suddenly I would get fatigued. I want to say tired, but it was different than being tired or sleepy. It was like all the energy had drained from my body and I had to lie down before I fell out of my chair.

It wasn't like I would fall asleep once I hit the couch. It was more like I would black out for an hour or so. I'd come to, lying on my back, our cat Champagne—a lovely champagne colored kitten—sitting on my chest purring away. It was like she knew I wasn't well and that I needed the company. It was kind of sweet, actually.

At that point, I finally made an appointment to see my doctor.

My doctor ran all the standard tests—blood pressure, heart, ear, nose and eyes, reflexes and he sent me for blood work. A couple of weeks later I went back to see my doctor. Everything looked good, he said. So he decided to send me to see a neurologist who examined me and sent me for an MRI.

I also had various blood tests and an evoked potential test. A spinal tap was suggested but I managed to squirm out of it. I have a thing about needles and the idea of having one stuck in my spine tapping me the way one taps a maple tree for sap made me go weak at the knees. Besides, the other tests ruled out pretty much everything, so I was allowed to skip the spinal tap. (I'm not saying that if your neurologist suspects that you have MS you should skip the spinal tap. Depending on the results of your other tests, you might need it to rule out other diseases.)

While I was initially diagnosed with RRMS, I may now have SPMS as my current symptoms have not gone into remission over the last four years. However, there is a reason my neurologist won't officially diagnose me with SPMS: my brain lesions have not gotten any larger in my last two MRIs. Suffice it to say we are playing the wait-and-see game. But it's been a long wait, and we haven't seen any improvements in my health in quite some time.

Freaking Out Over MS Diagnosis

I freaked out over my MS diagnosis. I was not an MS Warrior then.

I had a wife and seven-year-old daughter, Kyah, and no life insurance, and I thought I was going to die. I'm sure the neurologist explained that I wasn't going to drop dead, but it felt like I had just been handed a death sentence.

I remember that I was sitting on the couch with Lyn. I think we were both in tears. My exact words to her were this: "You might as well dig a hole and bury me."

I was barely forty. I was angry. I was depressed. I was scared. I thought it best that Lyn get rid of me and get on with her life. To her credit, she called me an idiot and did not take my advice. And look at me, twenty years later: cool as the proverbial cucumber. Suffice it to say, I still have MS. I still don't like the fact that I have it. I still sure as hell wish I didn't have it. I know it's not going to go away. I think though that it is fair to say that my attitude has changed.

But in those early days…

The first attack lasted just over a year. Symptoms went away for two years, and then returned, and I was officially diagnosed with MS, as opposed to possible MS.

Lyn asked if I would mind if she talked about what I was going through with some of her friends. Initially I said "no!" I didn't want people knowing what I was dealing with. Perhaps I was embarrassed or ashamed by MS. It took me a while to figure out two important aspects of this disease: one, it wasn't my fault that I had it; two, I may have had the disease, but Lyn was going through my illness with me. She needed to talk to people about how she was feeling too. So one day in a moment of enlightenment, I told her to talk away about anything to anybody. I had gotten over the hump of feeling embarrassed and ashamed and of feeling sorry for myself. And guess what? The sky did not fall.

In short, MS (and any chronic illness) is something you need to talk about. Not ad nauseam. That just gets boring and tedious. But in an informative and constructive manner at an appropriate time with appropriate people.

With that in mind, here is what else I've gotten to talk about.

The Eyes Have It

One night, when I looked up at street lights I saw halos. It was as if I was looking at angels in medieval paintings. You know the figures with the golden halos around their heads. That's what I saw when I looked into the lights. I wasn't squinting to make it happen. It was just happening. During the day, there was no real problem, although reading books, magazines and newspapers had become difficult. Ironically, I was able to read well on my computer. This was a relief as I am a writer and I spend all day in front of the computer screen.

Of course, most sane people would probably rush of to a doctor the day after such a phenomenon occurred. Me? I just continued to stare at street lights and make halos appear. I did this for a month or so and then one night the halos simply disappeared. However, that was not the end of the eye issues.

A few months later, I was driving my car down a residential street near our house and turned my head slightly in one direction. There are four-way stop signs at almost every intersection on the street and what I noticed, or didn't notice, disturbed me. I didn't notice the expected stop sign. I turned my head in another direction and the stop sign materialized.

I kept my eyes straight ahead until I got home. The rest of the stop signs all showed up, as they should have. Once I parked the car I played with moving my head about. I noticed there was a black spot over my right eye. I could literally black out signs, windows, cars, the heads of people—you name it—by looking at them with my right eye.

I went to see my doctor. He ran a few tests and booked an appointment for me with an eye specialist. A week or so later, the eye doctor saw me. He examined my eyes and ran a few tests. He booked an appointment for me to come back a week later. When I returned he explained that I had some sort of eye astigmatism and that it would never go away. He said it had always been there but was only manifesting itself due to age and the weakening of my retina. He booked a returned visit for three months later, just for the heck of it I guess.

Two weeks before I was due to see the eye doctor again, the stigma that was to never go away went away. It just vanished. I called the doctor's office and explained this to his assistant. We cancelled the appointment. She said to book a new appointment if the black spot ever returned. It's been fifteen years. It's never returned.

Why do I now think that this was an MS exacerbation? Since those two strange eye things (as you can see, I'm up on my medical terminology) I've had hits that have been formally diagnosed as exacerbations. I've also talked to a lot of people with MS. They have had similar eye things, known more formally as optic neuritis.

I've said it before, I'll say it again: what a strange disease is MS.

Tastes Like...

The next hit, when it came, was almost funny. Yet in some ways it was also the worst one I've experienced, until the headaches that plague me now.

My next hit was to my (drum roll, please)... taste buds! I didn't lose my taste. That would have been a blessing in comparison to what happened. What happened was this: everything that I tasted, tasted liked crap. Okay, I've never actually tasted crap, so let me qualify that. Everything that I tasted, tasted like what I imagine crap must taste like.

When I say everything, I mean everything. Give me a glass of water and I'd say, "Did you draw this water from a polluted swamp?" It was that bad.

To her credit, Lyn tried to tease my taste buds back into shape. She gave me salty foods, sweet foods, lemony foods, bland foods—all trying to discover if there was something that would taste okay or at least not so bad, to no avail.

I think I lost about thirty pounds while my taste buds were wonky, not that I couldn't stand to lose a few pounds.

To make a long taste story short, after about six months, my skunky taste retreated and all was fine.

The taste hit was one of the weirdest MS exacerbations that I have experienced. However, I hate my current condition—my 24/7 headaches. If I got to chose, I'd pick the crappy taste over the headaches. That's how much I'd appreciate some relief from what ails me now.

While coping with my current condition, I have learned to take pleasure in walking our dog, reading good books (or at least decent page-turners), watching good (mostly British) TV and playing interactive tablet games like Words with Friends (hey, if you play it look me up and challenge me; I'm not an expert by any stretch, but I do okay) and Yahtzee with Buddies.

The neurologist has prescribed two different drugs and a vitamin cocktail to try to combat the headaches. But nothing has helped.

We have also discussed various medications that are supposed to combats MS lesions—limit their growth and spread. I confess, I do not like the potential side effects of the drugs we discussed, especially the ones that could, potentially, damage the liver. I mean I figure it is bad enough that I am dealing with MS. I don't want to deal with liver damage too.

Just so you know, I am not anti-drug for the sake being anti-drug. I am just cautious. If I could find a drug that got rid of my headaches, I'd take it! In addition, I don't advocate that everybody with MS take the non-medical route. Doing so sure as hell has not cured me. But then there ain't no cure for MS. I am just getting on with life as best I can. It's a different life than it has been, but life can be lived, even with MS.

It's Friendship

As for friends, I used to go to monthly lunches with a writers' group. I don't any more. The group still meets, and I am still invited to join in. I just don't have the energy to get off my butt and socialize. One of the writers from the group drops by every now and then with muffins and we have a nice chat. Another has recently got a puppy and I see her once in a while when walking our Giant Schnauzer. We always have a nice chat and I was recently happy to pass on a writing job to her that I didn't have the energy to take on. But the sad fact is that I'm just not as social as I used to be.

We have good friends who come over for dinner once or twice a month. Sometimes Lyn cooks; sometimes we order in. They always bring a great fruit salad for dessert. I've known them since high school so if they are over and I get tired I'm comfortable sitting on the couch, putting my head back and closing my eyes for ten minutes until my second wind kicks in. Same when Kyah and her partner or my sister and her partner come over: I can be my MS self. But let's face it, that's not how you typically socialize.

I go to some of Lyn's family events. It depends on how I am feeling. When I go, I eat my meal and then sit on the couch and commiserate with Lyn's niece who is combating postural orthostatic tachycardia syndrome (POTS). We compare symptoms and treatments, and basically bore the heck out of anybody who happens to be sitting nearby.

I confess, there are days I wonder if what I am feeling is MS or if I'm just getting older. After all, I turn 65 this year. I know people age at different rates, but technically people don't retire until they 65. I couldn't teach or train in person if my life depended on it. (I can teach online writing webinars, but I limit them to two-hour sessions as opposed to the full-day workshops I used to conduct.) Also, while Lyn might have occasional aches that people our age have, she has way more energy than I have (understatement).

Simply put, there are things that I don't do anymore due to my MS. Can I do them? Some of them, perhaps. But I'd have to dig really deep to find the energy. I'd be uncomfortable doing them, and I'd pay for having done them. And many things I am simply unable to do.

I guess what I am saying is that my MS makes me feel like I am aging prematurely and more rapidly than I should be aging. But hey, I know that people get sick from many things. And others have long, healthy lives. So I am not complaining, not really, about what has happened to me. I am just trying to cope with it as best I can. And so is my wife, bless her warm, loving, generous soul.

MS is the hand I've been dealt. I don't have to like it. But it seems to me that I have no choice but to play it. Doesn't mean I am going to win; doesn't mean I am going to lose. Playing the hand we are dealt is what we all do as we go through this strange thing called life.

If you have any other suggestion about how to deal with it, feel free to email me-- msandmebook@gmail.com. Whether you agree or disagree with me, whether you think I'm nuts or sane. I have nothing to lose by listening to you. And I may even reply. After all, I seem to have a certain amount of MS induced time on my hands.

20 / Two Other Warriors Write

Two other MS Warriors have contributed essays to this book. Good to have other voices address topics that are outside of my range of experience. I am happy to turn the pages over to them.

A Complicated Option: MS Clinical Trials for Research

by Alicia Rasley

Paul asked me to write about my experience with MS. Short story: diagnosed 12 years ago at 48, worst flare-up was the first very bad one. Started treatment immediately. Now in long-term remission with a few remaining symptoms. But also have thoughts on "Big Pharma," that is, the huge international pharmaceutical companies that research, develop, and sell treatments for conditions like MS.

Now I have to say, MS is a disease practically designed for Big Pharma, as it utilizes their strengths—the ability and skill to spend literally decades researching different aspects of the disease, and access to huge funding and large populations of patients. Also, frankly, MS is a disease that is much more common in developed countries with health insurance, research universities, and medical infrastructure, which means that there's a big financial payoff for the companies that develop effective MS drugs.

For those reasons, most of the huge pharmaceutical companies have been testing treatments for MS since the first great advance in 1992 (interferon). I know most everyone hates Big Pharma, but really, this experience has been good for me, and I can't argue with that reality now. When I was first diagnosed, I predicted I'd be in a wheelchair or dead by this point. And I'm pretty much okay, especially considering how long I've had this crippling disease.

When I was diagnosed in 2006, I was self-employed and poorly insured. I still remember the first phone call I had with the pharmacist about what the then-standard treatment cost: $2,000 a month. I'm afraid I let slip a few shocked cuss words, as that was more than my entire salary. But a friend of a friend of a friend had also just been diagnosed and passed on a tip—researchers all over the world were conducting "clinical trials" of various drugs, and I should try to get into one of those trials to get free medication.

My mother was a biochemist who conducted research into botulism and salmonella (food-poisoning), so I am more comfortable than most with labs and white coats and test tubes. And while I'm not naïve about "Big Pharma." I know what important work researchers like my mother did in preventing and mitigating disease all through the 20th Century.

Fortunately, there were several medical schools doing clinical trials in my regions. I have to admit that I chose the first clinical trial because it was taking place at my alma mater (University of Chicago). Fortunately, I happened into a good trial. There was nothing very experimental or scary going on. The researcher (a neurology professor) was comparing the standard dose of the standard treatment with a double dose of the standard treatment. That is, the drug had already been tested and approved by the FDA, and the relative safety was established. (Most MS drugs fool around with the immune system, so none of them are completely harmless.)

I drove up to Chicago to be tested every month for years, and left each time with a few boxes of the syringes with the medication. While this was no cure, my condition stopped deteriorating so rapidly. And of course, I did my little bit to advance medical science knowledge of MS. When that clinical trial ended, I knew more of what made a clinical trial good for a patient, and chose the next one very wisely.

So if you're considering using clinical trials to get free meds, here are some considerations:

1. Make sure it's a "medications" trial. There are many different types of trials, looking at surgical options, lifestyle changes, and so on. Those might all be useful—I've been in a few "applied health" trials testing lifestyle modifications—but those won't get you medications. Medication trials are usually conducted by medical researchers with MDs, and held at research universities with teaching hospitals.

2. Try to get a "Phase 4" study. This is the phase where the basic efficacy of the medication has already been established. In this phase, you're unlikely to be put into a control group that receives a placebo (that is, no medication), because the placebo phase will already be completed. You'll be getting either a standard medication or the drug under study.

3. Talk through the requirements of the study before you sign on. These trials can last years. (The last one I was in is in its seventh year.) Will it fit with your lifestyle and health? I was a pretty perfect subject for a long-term trial because I am not going to move away from the trial location, and my job lets me go in for the frequent test appointments and follow ups. But parents of young children, workers with demanding jobs, or small businesspersons might not be able to commit to the appointment schedule. You can of course drop out of a trial at any point, but the longer you can commit, the better for both you and the trial.

4. Make sure treatment is provided free of charge for you. In fact, there is usually some reimbursement for expenses (usually less than $100 a visit).

5. Understand that the researcher is NOT your clinician. While the researcher should let you know when there's any risk or when blood tests show something wrong, he/she shouldn't treat you but refer you to another colleague. It's all very complicated, the role of the researcher to the patient, but at best, you should keep your own family doctor and a neurologist you can consult as needed.

6. Clinical trials often have restrictive requirements, such as that you not undertake other "competing" treatments and that you keep the researcher completely aware of any medications or supplements you're taking. Some quite common drugs (like statins) can have an effect on MS (potentially positive, in the case of statins), so they want to keep track of what else you're taking to account for that variation. Be open about drug and alcohol use also.

7. There are always risks to any treatment, and by law the researchers are required to communicate these to you. The "miracle drug" I was last tested on had a side effect of interfering with the thyroid gland, and I ended up having to take Synthroid for the rest of my life. (It isn't completely clear that this happened because of the treatment—thyroid disease is common in women over 50 already.) Talk over the risks with your research team and your family and decide how big a risk is too big (1%? 10%?) balanced against the expected rewards.

8. Being in a clinical trial means you are giving up options. You don't get to choose what group you get into, or what medication or dosage you get. This wasn't a problem when I first got started. As there were so few MS drugs then, it wasn't like we patients had much choice. Now there are a dozen approved treatments, and more coming every year. Fortunately, most of the medications are still under study, so if you think Tysabri, for

example, is the best treatment for you, you can probably find a trial researching that drug.

9. One great benefit of a clinical trial is access to cutting-edge information about the latest MS research. Another is near-constant monitoring of your health, as you get vitals and blood taken at almost every visit. It was my research nurse, for example, who alerted me to the fact that my pre-hypertension was getting worse.

Every MS patient has a different path to walk, and I would never want to interfere with another's choices. But if you are considering medication, and especially if you can't afford it or your insurance won't pay for it, you might check out clinical trials. The NARCOMS Registry for Multiple Sclerosis research (www.narcoms.org) and the US Government registry of clinical trials (clinicaltrials.gov) are good places to get started. And Health Talk (www.healthtalk.org/peoples-experiences/medical-research/clinical-trials/what-are-clinical-trials-and-why-do-we-need-them) is an exploration of the considerations involved in getting started in a clinical trial.

As for my experience, well, it's been a mixed blessing. (I've endured literally hundreds of blood draws). The last clinical trial I was in was the most arduous, for Lemtrada (which is usually used for lymphoma) with a two-year infusion (IV) treatment. I've been in remission (and off all medication) for five years now. I don't know what the future will hold, of course, but if my condition starts to deteriorate, I know I have clinical options, and now I have contacts with the best researchers in the country. And I feel like I have contributed at least a little to medical research in honor of my mother, Dr. Jeanne Todd. I think she would approve of my participation!

Alicia Rasley is an award-winning novelist who teaches writing at the University of Maryland and in workshops around the country. If you're interested in writing a novel or memoir, check out The Story Journey website (www.aliciarasley.com) for lots of free writing advice.

* * * * *

Thanks, Alicia. That was a breath of fresh air compared to my often frosty attitude towards drugs. There is no denying it, different people have different reactions to different drugs. That is simply one of many reasons that I call MS the Snowflake Disease. It is also why I suggest that MS Warriors discuss their options with their medical care givers and make informed choices. Don't expect miracle cures, but be hopeful and monitor the results, positive or (hopefully not) negative of any drug you take. Adapt as may be necessary.

And now another MS Warrior writes.

Tania Granger has her Titans to help her combat MS

By Tania Granger

I was diagnosed with MS in late 2010 after an MRI for back pain I'd been dealing with since my teen years. A few short months later, I started an interferon medication to help slow the disease's progress. I was 38 years old, had been married to my husband Dan for 10 years and had two children, Ben, who had just turned nine, and Emma, six. My determination was completely focused on raising my children before this disease touched me physically. I had a lot to be grateful for, but my health was taking a completely unexpected turn.

When my youngest was about three, I started heading to a local gym, and that led to a love of running. Because of my back issues I had to take it easy, but the day I ran my first 5K race with my husband, I sobbed at the finish. To this day, it's one of my greatest accomplishments.

Following my diagnosis in 2010, I registered a group of friends that I called "Tania's Titans" in a 5K Walk for MS that would take place the following summer. I remember seeing an advertisement for an MS Bike event. I was wishing I was healthy and fit enough to be able to participate. There was no way my back pain would allow for that to be even remotely possible.

But two years, and two MS walks later, I registered for my first MS Bike event in 2014—a two-day return journey between Ottawa and Cornwall that would involve between 80 and 215 km of riding, by myself. My husband, although proud, thought I was crazy.

I trained hard, ate well, and tried to rest as best as I could. I had never been so excited to do anything so intense and physically demanding. I answered all the questions swirling around in my mind with: "One kilometre at a time; one pit stop at a time."

My friends and family were excited and nervous for me and the messages I received while prepping for the ride were overwhelming. I packed up my bike and my gear and headed for Ottawa the night before the ride. Dan and the kids were driving to Cornwall on Day One of the event to provide support. It was so exciting, and I felt so proud to be able to teach my kids how to react when faced with a challenge. They met me at the finish following the first 125K and followed me back to the start line in Ottawa, which became the finish line on Day Two, and were there to see me cross the finish. I DID IT!

The motivation I feel from joining an event, either alone or with a team helps me mentally deal with living with this disease. It gives me the hope that I need to keep myself healthy and active so I can continue to participate year after year. My Tania's Titans team has participated in two local MS Walks and seven MS Bike events. We are gearing up for this year's Ottawa-Cornwall event. I have a group of more than 20 amazing friends and family who have joined me for one, two, or more events and together have helped raise almost $30,000 for the MS Society of Canada. That includes barbecues, yard sales, bake sales, raffles, and other events to help raise money for the events.

Nerve ablation treatments at the Kingston Orthopaedic Pain Institute have been successful in terms of back pain. I have been able to gain enough physical strength because of my determination (and an amazing trainer) to be able to participate in events like a half marathon and the "Tough Mudder" event.

I am staying optimistic and using "the power of positive thinking" to help me deal with the day-to-day stresses of this disease.

If I do everything right the majority of the time, then I'll have nothing to kick myself for, wishing I'd done things differently or avoiding the "I should've" attitude when reflecting on the past. It's been eight years since being diagnosed and I'm healthier now than I was then. Eating a healthy diet, keeping my immune system calm, and working with my Titans help keep me going!

This year's Ottawa-Cornwall MS Bike: Gear Up to End MS is being held August 18 and 19. Here's a link — goo.gl/QjsPQU — to the MS website where you can donate to help me end MS.

Tania Granger
Napanee, ON

* * * * *

Thanks, Tania, for letting us know about what you are doing to help combat MS. I applaud your effort to raise funds for the cure by walking and cycling, and for getting your "Titans" involved with your efforts.

I confess, I am a tad jealous too. I used to love to ride my bike. I'd ride it for hours and hours, travelling to all ends of the city (Toronto). I still remember the day when riding up a street on a minor incline to get home became an effort. At first I thought I was getting old. But heck, forty-five is not old. I know now it was MS weakening my legs. A while after I struggled to make it up the incline—and it really was not steep—I had to give up riding my bike all together. I could no longer cycle anywhere. As I've said, I can still walk my dog, and do so diligently. But I sure miss riding my bike.

Again, Tania, I applaud what you do and how you do it!

20 / Missing Aspects of Life

When I had RRMS, there were many months, several years even, when life was fine. I was in remission and could do whatever I needed to do—work, play, travel. There were even times when my exacerbations did not prevent me from working or doing stuff. After all, if your exacerbation is a hit to the taste buds, you can still get things done. You might not enjoy your food, but other than that your MS is not preventing you from living your life as you want to live it.

Today, simply put, there are things that I don't do anymore due to my MS. Can I do them? Some, perhaps. But I'd have to dig deep to find the strength and energy. I'd be uncomfortable doing them, and I'd pay for having done them. And there are many things I am simply unable to do.

I miss going out. I have no energy to dine out or go to a movie or to go out and watch my daughter do stand-up comedy or improv. Thank goodness for streaming on large screen TV sets!

What you can and cannot do is different for all of us with MS. I am not the only person with MS who misses stuff that we used to do. I asked on several MS support groups what people missed since being diagnosed with MS. The replies came in fast and furious.

"I miss running, or just moving quickly."

"I miss working. I was just diagnosed, and I'm not sure how all this will affect me."

"I miss working, exercise and generally helping people."

"Laying by the pool or going to the lake. The heat brings back previous flare ups almost instantly."

"I miss going for walks."

"Knitting. I can no longer knit. My left hand cramps up painfully when I hold the left needle."

"I miss walking with no cane."

"I had to change my diet. I miss fast food and donuts."

"Swimming. That's what I miss."

"Going to the river in the summer with our boat. It gets hot there and it just knocks me on my ass."

"I miss just walking about, without thinking about it."

"Having the energy to do things."

"I used to work. Now… Well, suffice it to say I no longer work."

"I miss remembering what I need to or want to do."

"I miss the strength to walk the cliffs and coastline."

"Playing roller derby. Running with ease, too. Oh, the stuff I took for granted!"

"I miss going for walks and bike rides. I miss exercising and playing softball and I miss dancing and high-heel shoes. But I am thankful for what I can still do!"

"I miss being able to run around the playground with my daughter."

"Driving at night."

"Driving. I'd be like a drunk behind the wheel."

"Friends. Where did they all go?"

"I miss being able to be with family without feeling like they feel sorry for me. I love that they care, I just hate feeling like I'm being pitied. And I'm not sure how to tell them that it bothers me."

"I can't ski anymore, or run, or even play hop scotch."

"Dancing!"

"Walking. The wheelchair keeps me mobile, except when it snows, but oh what I'd pay to feel my feet on the ground again."

"Happiness."

"Living."

So, as you can see, what we miss is different for each of us with this bizarre disease. The question is this: Are you going to pine for the life you had? I don't moan about what I miss. I miss it, but I don't moan and complain about it. Because pining, moaning and complaining won't change a thing. I simply try to make the most of life as it is.

What I am saying is this: if you are sick it is your job to try to find your new life within the limitations of your new reality. You don't have to believe me or adopt my philosophy. However, allow me to ask you this: What else are you going to do? How else are you going to live? I am not saying you have to, or should, like what MS has done to you. I am saying you don't need to let MS define you. You don't need to let MS win.

For instance, I am writing this book in short energetic bursts. Because that is what I can do. I can no longer conduct writing workshops in person or teach classes in person. Instead, I conduct online business and promotional writing webinars and teach online continuing education writing courses. I walk my dog, often twice a day. I don't walk as far as I did with my previous dog, but I still get out there with him, and my cane. I sell my business and promotional writing books online (www.paullima.com/books). I read more books than I used to and watch more TV shows and movies. But I look for good books to read and good shows to watch. In short, I do what my illness allows me to do.

I am not saying that you have to overcome your limitations. Limitations are, by definition, limitations. They limit what you can do. But I am also not saying that you should not strive to overcome them or at least live as full a life as you can live within their boundaries. I am saying you need to understand that you may have limitations, and you may have to find your new, post-MS life within them. And, I suggest, you need to plan for the future.

Plan for the Future

How do you plan for the future if you have such a fickle illness? I could say that you don't, but why wouldn't you plan for the future, at least as well as anybody else would—or better than others would! I can hear my financial planner friends shouting right now. "Of course you would plan for the future!" they'd say. "Who wouldn't?" In other words, you don't plan for the future just because you are ill. You plan for the future because it makes sense!

While I believe you have to live in the now, not constantly worrying and fretting about the future, I also feel you should plan for the future. Ironically, planning for it will reduce the amount of worrying and fretting you do in the now. I know that planning for the future when you are ill is kind of like juggling with fire and ice and razor blades and wet bars of soap. It's not easy, but it's what I suggest you try your best to do.

How we plan for the future will be different for each of us, kind of like this disease, depending on our health, age, relationship status, if we are able to work or not, if we have benefits and/or health insurance, if we have a support network of family and friends.

For instance, if you are relatively healthy now and working. Good on you. May I suggest you do your best to build a nest egg to support yourself in the future as may be required? If you have a partner who is working at a stable job with benefits, you may not have to squirrel away as much as someone with MS who is on their own, but you will still want to think about life down the road.

I am not being a pessimist here. I am not saying great ills will befall you. I am being a realist. Great ills will befall some of us with MS, just as they will befall a certain percentage of the population that does not have MS. So do what you can do to plan for your future, while living in your now.

If like me you are not terribly knowledgeable about all this planning for the future stuff, seek professional advice from a reliable financial planning source. But do try to alleviate some of your future concerns so that you can more fully live in a more relaxed present day—with future worries as alleviated as possible.

I know, more easily said than done, but do what you can do!

20 / MS Is Not A Death Sentence

Recent research in the United States indicates that people with MS may live an average of about seven years less than the general population because of various medical complications and because of how the exacerbations add up over the years. However, paying attention to overall health and wellness can help many people with MS live as long as others live. (That's right, you may want to rethink your beer and pretzels diet.) So MS is not a death sentence.

On the other hand, studies have also indicated that fifteen years following diagnosis, those with MS had a forty percent probability of needing some form of walking assistance and a twenty-five percent probability of being in a wheelchair. Some people with MS need walkers or canes to move down the street. Some people limp along. And some amble along quite nicely. It is the nature of the disease.

Some who amble quite nicely have cognitive impairments. Some people have visual impairments. Some of us experience strange sensations to different part of our bodies. Some of us experience strange sensations to almost every part of our bodies. We experience tremors, tingles, shakes, shooting pains.

Some of us go downhill from day one. Some of us go up and down, with periods of downs of various lengths followed by periods of ups of various lengths.

Some of us are on medications that help and have no side effects. Some of us are on medications that don't help and have minor, or major, side effects. Some of us are on medications that help and have minor, or major, side effects.

For some of us, dietary change has proven to be beneficial; for other it has not. And some of us, too few of us, become fine and stay that way for a long time.

I could go on, but I think you get the picture.

If You Want a Good Cry...

If you have MS and want a good cry (and I think people with MS should have a good cry every now and then) watch the movie *100 metros* (*100 Metres*). It is based on the true story of a Spanish man with MS who trains for an Iron-Man competition: 3.8 km swimming, 180 km cycling and 42 km running. He is told by his doctors that he'd be lucky if he could make 100 metres, hence the name of the film. I don't want to give too much away, but as he is training for the competition he has to halt his training because he has a relapse. He has RRMS, which means he should go into remission at some point too, no? But you will have to watch the movie (subtitled) to see what happens. All I'll say is it is well worth viewing. (As of the writing of this book it was streaming on Netflix.)

SPOILER ALERT: If you hate spoilers please move down a couple of paragraphs, after the second set of asterisks.

* * *

I'm going to tell you how the movie ends. It's still worth watching. Trust me.

Our main character completes the Iron-Man competition. It takes him all day, but he completes it. I suspect if he didn't complete it there would be no movie. He remains MS symptom free for three years, and then he relapses. And let us face it, one day this MS Iron-Man Warrior will pass away, as will we all. Death. It is inevitable. The question is this: Will you complete your Iron-Man competition before you pass away?

I consider this book the second stage of my Iron-Man competition. The first stage was my book, *MS & ME: From First Signs, To Diagnosis, To Living With Chronic Illness* (paullima.com/books). *MS & ME* chronicles my 20 years of dealing with MS and I have incorporated important aspects of me and my version of MS into this book, so I am not trying to sell it to you!

If you are reading this book, then I have completed the second stage and have one more stage to go. Other I hope I have many more stages to go. Wish me luck. And watch the movie. Then pick your Iron-Man Competition equivalent and start to train for it.

* * *

With my mini movie review, and spoiler, out of the way, allow me to say that I don't want to downplay just how sick people with MS can get. It can be a freaking debilitating disease. But allow me to be optimistic for a moment, even if it doesn't seem like that is how I am being off the top.

I know several people with MS who are in wheelchairs and several who use walkers. Others I know use canes, as do I. Others I know have various physical and cognitive impairments. At the same time, I know people with MS who are, how shall I put this? Who are all but fine. Perhaps even fine.

For instance, I know someone with MS who works fulltime, rides her bicycle everywhere and goes to the gym daily. She has been diagnosed with MS and experiences occasional cramping in her legs. That is not to say she won't experience other MS symptoms down the line. That is to say she is fine right now. To her I say, "Live in the now." Why would she live any place else? Why would she give up her life worrying about the fact that her MS might flare up down the road, and that she might have to halt her equivalent of training for her Iron Man?

I know someone with MS who drives a cab. He is married and has two teenage children. He has been diagnosed with MS and experiences occasional tremors and some odd, unexplained nervousness. He tends to vape (a way of ingesting marijuana) in the evening as it calms him down and helps him sleep. (He never vapes before or while driving his cab. Never, ever.) That is not to say he won't experience other MS symptoms down the line. That is to say he is fine right now. To him I say, "Live in the now." Why would he live any place else? Why would he give up his life worrying about the fact that his MS might flare up down the road, and that he might have to halt his equivalent of training for his Iron Man?

I know someone with MS who dropped out of university. He has mild cognitive impairment. When I asked him if he regrets dropping out of university, he laughs. "Hell no. I hated the program that I was in!" He is a struggling artist. When I ask him if he attributes his artistic struggles to his MS, he laughs. "Hell no, I struggled with my art long before my diagnosis." He is looking for direction in life while dealing with his MS. That is not to say he won't experience other MS symptoms down the road. That is to say he is fine right now, other than being a bit at loose ends. To him I say, "Live in the now." Why would he live any place else? Why would he give up his life worrying about the fact that his MS might flare up down the road, and that he might have to halt his equivalent of training for his Iron Man?

That is not to say that MS can't be debilitating. Sadly, and most unfortunately, it can be.

If you have PPMS the reality is that you will most likely end up in a wheelchair. You most likely will even start to lose the functions of your arms and hands, in addition to your legs, as time progresses.

My heart aches for you. We both have MS, but I cannot image how such symptoms must feel. At the same time, and I am not downplaying what you may go through, you will not end up in a wheelchair the day after, week after, month after or even year after you are diagnosed with MS. You will have time to live your life and, most important, time to adapt to MS as best you can. And I know people in wheel chairs who adapted well to their MS.

Again, I am not trying in any way to downplay what can be, and too often are, devastating effects of this disease. I am trying to say that for most of us with MS, life goes on. Yes, we and our loved ones, have to adapt to what MS brings on. It's kind of like growing old prematurely and at a more rapid rate that we otherwise would do if we were healthy. But we would have to deal with growing older even if we were healthy.

The fact is this: MS is not a death sentence. It is a barrier. An impediment. An obstacle. It is something you need to learn how to live with, and overcome when and if you can, because, even if it is different for each of us, it is never going to go away.

How many healthy people do you hear complain about impediments, barriers and obstacles? When you were healthy, how many times did you face them? Fact is, people who are healthy and have healthy attitudes face their limitations head on, and overcome them.

You may be ill, but your attitude can be healthy. You can face the impediments, barriers, obstacles—the challenges—that MS, that life, puts in your way. What are your options? Roll up into a ball? Put your head in the sand? Or face the impediments, barriers and obstacles head on as best you can given your MS limitations?

Your goal is to succeed, and to succeed as often as you can. But guess what? You are going to fail at times? So what? So do healthy people.

I guess what I am saying is the real goal is to try and to keep on trying, no matter what. No matter how challenging. No matter how daunting. No matter how painful. No matter how frustrating. No matter what.

Mic, a man with PPMS, a guy in a wheelchair and a real MS Warrior, had one of the healthiest MS attitudes I am aware of, and a great sense of humor. He had a saying, and you will excuse my one swear word in this book:

"Fuck MS!" he'd say.

In other words, this MS Warrior was not going to let MS defeat him. He worked damn hard, as he wheeled through life, to overcome the barriers, impediments and obstacles that MS put in his path. Others with MS loved him for it—for his inspiration and motivation.

Yes MS took him, at least contributed to his death, way too soon. But in the end life takes us all. It's what we do with life while we are here that matters. That counts.

So with all that in mind, some final thoughts.

Eat well. Stay fit. Adapt as best you can. See your neurologist. Find out about medications and their potential side effects. Make informed decisions about any medications you choose to take. Monitor for side effects. Maintain a positive attitude. But allow yourself to feel pissed off and angry now and then. But don't take your anger out on others who can support you. And don't blame yourself for this frustrating and infuriating disease. You've done nothing wrong. It has just happened to you. Adjust as best you can. Gather around as much support as you can, including in-person and/or online support groups.

Live as full a life as you can. You deserve it. Despite MS. You deserve as full a life as you can live. So live your life to the fullest.

21 / Epilogue

If you were to observe me from a distance, you'd probably say something like, "Paul looks pretty good. He's teaching online writing courses and webinars. He's writing a book. He walks his dog every day. He goes out for dinner now and then. He enjoys reading a good book and watching great television series. What's the problem?"

What you would not see is that I am doing all of what you have observed while feeling like crap. Constantly like crap.

You won't see that feeling because it is not on the outside. I'm not purple. I don't have any physical deformity. The feeling is all inside. It's my constant headaches. It's my constant vertigo-like dizziness. It's my loss of balance. It's my feet constantly feeling like they are on fire. It's my exhaustion.

These symptoms and more you don't see in MS Warriors, unless they need a walker or a scooter or a wheel chair to get around. I use a cane, you can see that. But if need be I can walk without it.

That is the nature of MS. MS is there, but out of sight. It is an invisible disease, as are many other diseases. So please don't think for a moment that I am saying that only MS Warriors have it bad! I am saying that MS is what I have to live with and deal with.

The fact that MS is out of sight might lead you to think that it is all in my head. And you'd be right. I have the MRI results that prove it. See those lesions in my MRI? Those lesion on my brain (and spinal cord and sometimes on my optic nerve). Those lesions in my head are my MS. So there it is, in my head.

I didn't ask for it. I sure as hell don't want it. But I have it.

What am I going to do with it? I can't think of anything to do, other than live with it to the best of my ability. So that is what I am doing, and that is what I am going to continue to do, even though I feel like crap constantly. I have no desire to roll up in a ball. I have no desire to just give up.

Oh, there are days, trust me, when I feel that way. Like giving up. There are days when I don't want to get out of bed. On those days, I take a deep breath, acknowledge the feeling, maybe even wallow in it for a bit. But then I unravel myself and get up and get on with it.

This book is an example of that. My life, I hope, is an example of that.

So now you know everything you need to know, or almost everything you need to know, about Multiple Sclerosis.

If you are an MS Warrior, I hope that your MS is benign, or at least as mild as possible. I wish you long periods of remission or a slow progression if remission is not possible. And I hope that this book, and any knowledge and understanding about your disease that you have gained from it, gives you some comfort as you progress through life with MS.

If you are a friend, family member or care giver of an MS Warrior, I hope that this book, and any knowledge and understanding you have gained from it, gives you some idea of what the MS Warrior in your life is going through, and why.

I guess for me that is the bottom line: *hope*. Hope for the best for all of us with this fickle and bizarre disease called MS.

21 / List of Online MS Resources

Here is a brief list of online MS resources and information. All links here are, as best as I can tell, legitimate resource that will not try to sell you any snake oil. Some may have links to legitimate fundraising efforts—nothing too overt—that you can, of course, choose to ignore, or not, depending on your mood and financial situation.

All the links listed here were active as of the writing of this book. You know what the Web is like: some of the links may have changed since I last checked them out.

- National Multiple Sclerosis Society (USA) - https://www.nationalmssociety.org/
- The Multiple Sclerosis Association Of America - https://mymsaa.org/
- Multiple Sclerosis Society of Canada - https://mssociety.ca/
- Latest in MS research presented at the 65th American Academy of Neurology Annual Meeting - https://mssociety.ca/research-news/article/latest-in-ms-research-presented-at-the-65th-american-academy-of-neurology-meeting
- What is MS - https://mssociety.ca/about-ms/what-is-ms
- Causes of MS symptoms - https://mssociety.ca/about-ms/symptoms
- Multiple sclerosis - Symptoms and causes - Mayo Clinic - https://www.mayoclinic.org/diseases-conditions/multiple-sclerosis/symptoms-causes/syc-20350269
- What is Multiple Sclerosis: https://www.webmd.com/multiple-sclerosis/what-is-multiple-sclerosis#1
- Multiple sclerosis - Wikipedia - https://en.wikipedia.org/wiki/Multiple_sclerosis
- Is Multiple Sclerosis (MS) Fatal? Symptoms, Treatment - MedicineNet - https://www.medicinenet.com/multiple_sclerosis_ms/article.htm
- Understanding Multiple Sclerosis: A Detailed Overview - Healthline - https://www.healthline.com/health/multiple-sclerosis
- Learn about MS with Aaron Boster MD (YouTube videos): https://www.youtube.com/c/AaronBosterMD
- Paul Lima's Me and My MS blog: https://mymsblogsite.wordpress.com/
- Go to www.google.ca/alerts and set up a Google Alert for "Multiple Sclerosis" or any topic related to it, such as "Multiple Sclerosis research" and receive an alert whenever anything new about your topic is posted online

In addition, here are links to several online MS support groups (active at the time I was writing this book). Do see if you can find an in-person support group in your area. The local chapter of your MS society or perhaps your local library might have such a list. If there is no in-person support group, or even if there is, you may want to check out these online support groups.

- myMSteam—the social network for those living with multiple sclerosis - https://www.mymsteam.com

- Ocrevus (MS medication) Facebook support group - https://www.facebook.com/groups/877992585700537/
- Multiple Sclerosis Support (Facebook) - https://www.facebook.com/groups/202971306407870/
- The Multiple Sclerosis Support Group (Facebook) - https://www.facebook.com/groups/1598134280453863/

Note: there are other Facebook MS support groups as a Facebook search will turn up.

- Online Support Groups : National MS Society page - https://www.nationalmssociety.org/Programs-and-Services/Programs/Online-Support-Groups
- Join a Local Support Group : National MS Society page - https://www.nationalmssociety.org/Resources-Support/Find-Support/Join-a-Local-Support-Group
- Support and Self-help Groups - MS of Canada page - https://mssociety.ca/support-services/programs-and-services/support-and-self-help-groups
- Healthline Online Multiple Sclerosis Support Groups page - https://www.healthline.com/health/multiple-sclerosis/support-groups#modal-close

About the Author

Based in Toronto, Ontario, Paul Lima (www.paullima.com) has worked as a writer and business-writing instructor for over 35 years. He has run a successful freelance writing, copywriting, business writing, and training business since 1988.

Additional books by Paul Lima

- Every Thing You Need To Know About Multiple Sclerosis: For MS Warriors, Their Family, Friends and Care Givers
- MS & ME: From First Signs, To Diagnosis, To Living With Chronic Illness
- Harness the Business Writing Process: E-mail, Letters, Proposals, Reports, Media Releases, Web Content
- Harness the Email Writing Process: How to Become a More Effective and Efficient Email Writer
- Fundamentals of Writing: How to Write Articles, Media Releases, Case Studies, Blog Posts and Social Media Content
- How to Write Web Copy and Social Media Content
- Copywriting That Works: Bright ideas to Help You Inform, Persuade, Motivate and Sell!
- How to Write Sales Letters and Email: Write direct response marketing material to inform, persuade and sell!
- Say it Right: How to Write Speeches and Presentations
- How To Write A Non-Fiction Book in 60 Days
- Produce, Price and Promote Your Self-Published Fiction or Non-fiction Book
- Everything You Wanted to Know About Freelance Writing - Find, Price, Manage Corporate Writing Assignments & Develop Article Ideas and Sell Them to Newspapers and Magazines
- Six-Figure Freelancer: How to Find, Price and Manage Corporate Writing Assignments
- Business of Freelance Writing: How to Develop Article Ideas and Sell Them to Newspapers and Magazines, Conduct Interviews and Write Article Leads
- The Query Letter: How to Sell Article Ideas to Newspapers and Magazines
- Unblock Writer's Block: How to face it, deal with it and overcome it. With over 70 writing exercises to get you started and keep you writing.
- (re)Discover the Joy of Creative Writing.
- How to Write Media Releases to Promote Your Business, Organization or Event
- Are You Ready For Your Interview? How to Prepare for Media Interviews. Prepare for interviews with print and broadcast reporters.
- Rebel in the Back Seat and other short stories

The above books are available in print and/or digital format: paullima.com/books.

www.ingramcontent.com/pod-product-compliance
Lightning Source LLC
Chambersburg PA
CBHW081722270326
41933CB00017B/3261